ceeding in

views

earch

Plans

Students

DATE DUE

Transforming Nursing Practice series

Transforming Nursing Practice is the first series of books designed to help students meet the requirements of the NMC Standards and Essential Skills Clusters for degree programmes. Each book addresses a core topic, and together they cover the generic knowledge required for all fields of practice.

Core knowledge titles
Series editor: Professor Shirley Bach, Head of the School of Health Sciences at the University of Brighton

Personal and professional learning skills titles
Series editors: Dr Mooi Standing, Independent Academic Consultant (UK and International) & Accredited NMC Reviewer and Professor Shirley Bach, Head of the School of Health Sciences at the University of Brighton

Mental health nursing titles
Series editors: Sandra Walker, Senior Teaching Fellow in Mental Health in the Faculty of Health Sciences, University of Southampton and Professor Shirley Bach, Head of the School of Health Sciences at the University of Brighton

You can find more information on each of these titles and our other learning resources at www.sagepub.co.uk. Many of these titles are also available in various e-book formats; please visit our website for more information.

Succeeding in
Literature Reviews and Research Project Plans
for Nursing Students
Second edition

Graham R Williamson
Andrew Whittaker

⑤SAGE | **Ⓜ LearningMatters**

Los Angeles | London | New Delhi
Singapore | Washington DC

Learning Matters
An imprint of SAGE Publications Ltd
1 Oliver's Yard
55 City Road
London EC1Y 1SP

SAGE Publications Inc.
2455 Teller Road
Thousand Oaks, California 91320

SAGE Publications India Pvt Ltd
B 1/I 1 Mohan Cooperative Industrial Area
Mathura Road
New Delhi 110 044

SAGE Publications Asia-Pacific Pte Ltd
3 Church Street
#10-04 Samsung Hub
Singapore 049483

Editor: Alex Clabburn
Development editor: Ellie Rivers
Production controller: Chris Marke
Project management: Swales & Willis Ltd, Exeter, Devon
Marketing manager: Tamara Navaratnam
Cover design: Wendy Scott
Typeset by: C&M Digitals (P) Ltd, Chennai, India
Printed by: CPI Group (UK) Ltd, Croydon, CR0 4YY

Library of Congress Control Number: 2014937808

British Library Cataloguing in Publication Data

A CIP record for this book is available from the British Library

ISBN 978-1-4462-8282-3
ISBN 978-1-4462-8283-0 (pbk)

At SAGE we take sustainability seriously. Most of our products are printed in the UK using FSC papers and boards. When we print overseas we ensure sustainable papers are used as measured by the Egmont grading system. We undertake an annual audit to monitor our sustainability.

Contents

About the authors

Dr Graham R Williamson is a Lecturer in Adult Nursing at the University of Plymouth. His clinical background is in acute medical nursing. His areas of teaching expertise are in evidence-based practice and research. His research interests concern supporting students in clinical practice.

Andrew Whittaker is a Senior Lecturer in the Faculty of Health and Social Care at London South Bank University. He has taught nursing students since the early 1990s and teaches research skills to undergraduate and postgraduate students. He has worked in adult and child mental health and was the director of a mental health voluntary organisation.

Foreword

Succeeding in Literature Reviews and Research Project Plans for Nursing Students enables readers to prepare for, organise, carry out and successfully complete a research proposal and/or literature review to demonstrate the graduate skills needed to be awarded a degree. It is therefore an essential book for all undergraduate pre-registration nursing students. The authors are experienced in teaching, supporting and supervising nursing students who are undertaking a research project/literature review and the writing style of the book reflects this. They recognise that this is likely to be the most demanding academic piece of work that students have to produce in becoming graduate nurses. Readers are encouraged to actively participate as they are guided through choosing a nursing topic, developing questions about it, accessing and critically reviewing research literature, considering ethical issues, proposing research where applicable, and writing up their literature review or research proposal. Case studies are used throughout the book helping to link theory to practice, and to show how vital research skills are for nurses to deliver clinically effective, evidence-based care. The authors also offer practical tips to help students focus on aims that they can realistically achieve, and how to avoid 'pitfalls' such as not backing up files or leaving 'writing up' until the last minute.

In the second edition of this invaluable book the authors have updated references and websites, and incorporated changes in response to the helpful feedback received. In doing so, they highlight the dynamic nature of nursing knowledge/skills and the need for lifelong learning. Like others in the Transforming Nursing Practice series this book addresses NMC Standards and Essential Skills Clusters to equip students for their responsibilities as registered nurses. In this respect it complements other books in the series, particularly: *Understanding Research for Nursing Students, Evidence-based Practice in Nursing, Critical Thinking and Writing for Nursing Students* and *Clinical Judgement and Decision Making for Nursing Students.*

Dr Mooi Standing
Series Editor

Acknowledgements

Andrew Whittaker would like to dedicate this book to Samantha on her eighteenth birthday. He would like to thank his mother, father and sister, Sally and her family, Joe, Lauren-Kate and Ben for their support and encouragement. He would like to thank Rebecca, Samantha, Lily and Jonathan, who have now got used to him continually writing. But most of all, he would like to thank his wife, Christina, and say that he's looking forward to more precious time together.

Andrew would like to thank his supportive colleagues at London South Bank University, Martyn Higgins, Iain Campbell-King, John Macdonough, Jill Yates, Andrea Colquhoun, Tirion Havard, Michelle Evans, Annabel Goodyer, Carl Chandra, Jo Rawles, Mary Saunders, Tom Wilks, Rohan Burke, Claire Felix and Ruth Watson. He has appreciated the support of staff at Learning Matters at Sage, particularly Eleanor Rivers, Alex Clabburn and Becky Taylor, who have always been helpful and encouraging. He would like to thank current and past students for their helpful comments and suggestions.

Artwork

The authors and publisher are grateful for permissions to reproduce the following artwork:

Figure 6.2: CONSORT 2010 flow diagram. Reproduced from Moher et al. (2010). Made available under the Wikimedia Creative Commons License via Wikipedia (see http://creativecommons.org/licenses/by/3.0 for terms and conditions).   116

Figure 7.1: Normal distribution curve. Adapted from an original graph by Jeremy Kemp (2 September 2005). Made available under the Wikimedia Creative Commons License via Wikipedia (see http://creativecommons.org/licenses/by-sa/3.0 for terms and conditions).   125

Figure 7.4: Confidence intervals containing point estimates. Adapted from an original graph by Sigbert (8 December 2008). Made available under the Wikimedia Creative Commons License via Wikipedia (see http://creativecommons.org/licenses/by-sa/3.0 for terms and conditions).   127

Figure 7.5: Scatterplot showing a strong positive correlation between age and wrinkles. Adapted from an original graph by Lars Aronsson (8 December

2008). Made available under the Wikimedia Creative Commons License via Wikipedia (see http://creativecommons.org/licenses/by-sa/3.0 for terms and conditions). 130

Figure 7.6: Forest plot showing confidence intervals, point estimates as black boxes and a summary measure in the larger diamond. Reproduced from an original graph by Jimjamjak (4 May 2010). Made available under the Wikimedia Creative Commons License via Wikipedia (see http://creativecommons.org/licenses/by-sa/3.0/deed.en for terms and conditions). Under the terms of the GNU licence the original must be made available to readers and this is available at http://upload.wikimedia.org/wikipedia/commons/f/f0/Generic_forest_plot.png. 132

Figure 8.1: Generic funnel plot. Reproduced from an original graph by Nousernamesleft (21 January 2008). Made freely available for any purpose under the Wikimedia Creative Commons License via Wikipedia (see http://commons.wikimedia.org/wiki/Main_Page for further information). 141

Figure 8.2: Funnel plot showing publication bias. Adapted from an original graph by Nousernamesleft (21 January 2008). Made freely available for any purpose under the Wikimedia Creative Commons License via Wikipedia (see http://commons.wikimedia.org/wiki/Main_Page for further information). 141

Figure 8.3: The Cochrane Collaboration logo. Used with permission from Nick Royle, CEO, the Cochrane Collaboration, Oxford, UK. The Cochrane Collaboration logo is a registered trademark of the Cochrane Collaboration. 144

Figure 10.1: Gantt chart for project planning. Adapted from an original diagram by Garry L Booker (8 October 2007) and released into the public domain via Wikipedia. Made available under the Wikimedia Creative Commons License via Wikipedia (see http://creativecommons.org/licenses/by-sa/3.0/deed.en for terms and conditions). 180

Every effort has been made to trace all copyright holders within the book, but if any have been inadvertently overlooked the publisher will be pleased to make the necessary arrangements at the first opportunity.

Introduction

This book is written for students of nursing who are developing the knowledge and skills to complete the research project plans and literature reviews which are increasingly components of their programmes, typically as third-year studies. While it is primarily aimed at students in their final year or level of study on an undergraduate degree, it will also be useful for students on postgraduate programmes with a research component, including those studying at Master's level. It would also assist students undertaking a range of social and healthcare courses in further education, including social workers, midwives, occupational therapists and other health and social care professionals for whom research, project planning and reviewing literature are essential elements. Experienced and qualified nurses, especially those undertaking postgraduate studies, will also be able to use this book for consultation, teaching and revision and to gain an insight into the expectations raised in nursing degree programmes.

Requirements for nurse education

Nurse education has undergone a major transformation over the last 20 years as programmes of study have moved into university settings. More recently, the Nursing and Midwifery Council (NMC) announced in 2009 that the requirements for entry to the professional register have changed so that new entrants have needed a degree from 2013, with withdrawal of diploma programmes. Degree programmes are at a higher level, with higher expectations and different skills required. This is reflected in the NMC *Standards for Pre-registration Nursing Education* (NMC, 2010a) as well as their Essential Skills Clusters (NMC, 2010b) and the Quality Assurance Agency (QAA, 2001) subject benchmarks for nursing. We refer extensively below to these NMC and QAA requirements to illustrate the extent to which the NMC as a professional regulatory body, and the QAA as the agency that reviews the quality and standards of higher education in universities, insist that nurses develop research and evidence-based practice skills. Taken as a whole, this book maps to these standards.

> ### NMC Standards for Pre-registration Nursing Education: Competency Framework
>
> The NMC (2010a) Competency Framework for undergraduate nursing indicates the following areas of generic importance to all nursing programmes in relation to research and evidence. (Each branch also has a range of statements in its branch-specific requirements.)
>
> *(continued)*

continued ....

Domain: Professional values

9. All nurses must appreciate the value of evidence in practice, be able to understand and appraise research, apply relevant theory and research findings in their work, and identify areas for further investigation.

Domain: Nursing practice and decision making

1. All nurses must use up-to-date evidence to assess, plan, deliver and evaluate care, communicate findings, influence change and promote health and best practice. They must make person-centred, evidence-based judgements and decisions, in partnership with others involved in the care process, to ensure high quality care. They must be able to recognise when the complexity of clinical decisions requires specialist knowledge and expertise, and consult or refer accordingly.

Essential Skills Clusters

The NMC Essential Skills Clusters (2010b) require a level of research literacy and skills with evidence.

Cluster: Organisational aspects of care

9. People can trust the newly registered graduate nurse to treat them as partners and work with them to make a holistic and systematic assessment of their needs; to develop a personalised plan that is based on mutual understanding and respect for their individual situation promoting health and well-being, minimising risk of harm and promoting their safety at all times.

By entry to the register

• Applies research-based evidence to practice.

16. People can trust the newly registered graduate nurse to safely lead, co-ordinate and manage care.

By entry to the register

• Bases decisions on evidence and uses experience to guide decision making.

20. People can trust the newly registered graduate nurse to select and manage medical devices safely.

• Works within legal frameworks and applies evidence-based practice in the safe selection and use of medical devices.

Cluster: Medicines management

41. People can trust the newly registered graduate nurse to use and evaluate up-to-date information on medicines management and work within national and local policy guidelines.

By the second progression point
- Accesses commonly used evidence-based sources relating to the safe and effective management of medicine.

By entry to the register
- Works within national and local policies and ensures others do the same.

Benchmark Statement for Health Care Programmes

The QAA (2001) Benchmark Statement for Health Care Programmes indicates that in nursing the following are important in relation to research and evidence.

A1 Professional autonomy and accountability

The award holder should be able to:
- contribute to the development and dissemination of evidence-based practice within professional contexts.

A4 Profession and employer context

The award holder should be able to:
- recognise the value of research and other scholarly activity in relation to the development of the profession and of patient/client care;
- recognise the need for changes in practice from best available evidence.

The study of nursing encompasses the following principle:
- the application of current knowledge and research to nursing practice across the health and illness continuum.

B2 Formulation of plans and strategies for meeting healthcare needs

The award holder should be able to:
- use evidence-based options to facilitate patient choice and inform nursing interventions.

B3 Practice

The award holder should be able to:
- conduct appropriate activities skilfully and in accordance with best/evidence-based practice;
- apply evidence-based knowledge to inform nursing care decisions.

C1 Knowledge and understanding

The award holder should be able to demonstrate:
- understanding of the key concepts of the disciplines that underpin the education and training of all healthcare professionals, and detailed knowledge of some of these. The latter would include a broad understanding of:

(Continued)

(Continued)

- health and social care philosophy and policy, and its translation into ethical and evidence-based practice.

C2 Associated skills

The award holder should be able to:

Information gathering
- seek out research-based evidence related to specific client groups;
- show an ability to gather and evaluate evidence and information from a wide range of sources;
- show an ability to use methods of enquiry to collect and interpret data in order to provide information that would inform or benefit practice.

Problem solving and data collection and interpretation
- analyse, interpret and assess the value of evidence to inform problem solving.

Information technology
- access healthcare research and literature databases.

Teaching, learning and assessment

Generic and enabling skills
Programmes should be designed to facilitate students' acquisition of effective communication skills, team working, problem solving, the use of IT, research methodology and critical reasoning.

B Principles and concepts: application

The award holder should be able to:
- demonstrate critical understanding of research-based knowledge and the application to practice;
- use relevant theoretical and research evidence to inform a comprehensive, systematic assessment of the physical, psychological, social and spiritual needs of patients, clients and communities;
- critically evaluate research findings and suggest changes to planned care;
- use appropriate research and other evidence to underpin nursing decisions that can be justified, even when made on the basis of limited information.

C Subject knowledge, understanding and associated skills

The award holder should be able to:
- demonstrate an understanding of research and other evidence and, where appropriate, apply findings to practice;
- critically evaluate research findings, suggest changes to practice and contribute to healthcare research to inform practice development.

Implications for students

Although nursing is a very practical occupation, this emphasis can be mistaken as a call for 'common sense' rather than 'book knowledge'. However, common sense can be used to justify a range of taken-for-granted assumptions that are often unspoken and can perpetuate poor practice when they go unchallenged. Instead, an internationally accepted development in healthcare decision making is to maintain a patient focus and integrate the best of research findings, theoretical and experiential knowledge to ensure care is based on up-to-date evidence and is appropriate for the patient's/client's needs. You will find this referred to as evidence-informed decision making, indicating how important evidence should be in the treatment and care of individual patients and clients. This approach is known as clinical effectiveness, and relies on evidence-based practice to ensure that research findings are robust.

This book concentrates on supporting you to develop the core skills required to complete the research project-planning and literature-reviewing components of your programmes, particularly at degree level. An action-oriented approach helps to facilitate evaluation and review of your practice. Case studies, reflecting a range of different practice settings, will be used throughout to enhance this process and to illustrate key points.

Book structure

This book contains four sections, with ten chapters. Section 1 is called *Getting started*, and contains one large chapter called *Getting started on your final-year project*. It provides an overview of literature reviews, project plans and dissertations, including useful information about why they are undertaken, some of the expectations that go along with them, and what they can give you in terms of transferable skills and benefits in practice. This chapter also looks at the role of research in your final-year project.

Section 2 is called *Planning and preparing for your final-year project*, and contains two chapters. Chapter 2 is *Planning and undertaking a literature review or documentary analysis*, which focuses on the 'how to' aspects of this, as well as offering some insights which will help you to appraise and use research to inform practice. Chapter 3 is *Planning your research proposal or dissertation* and, again, provides practical material on how this can best be achieved.

In Section 3, *Using and critiquing research for your final-year project*, there are five chapters, and these have been written with the emphasis on helping students decide which approaches to use as part of their research plans or proposals, with some insights into how different approaches might be assessed as part of a literature review. There is little on undertaking the methods *per se*, instead, the emphasis is on understanding them, with a focus on the 'how' and 'why' rather than the 'what'. The first chapter of Section 3, *Using and critiquing research methods: interviews and focus groups* (Chapter 4), contains material on interviews and focus groups. Chapter 5 contains material on *Analysing qualitative data*, and looks at a popular method called thematic analysis. Chapter 6, *Using and critiquing research methods: surveys and experimental designs*, has a focus on experimental designs and randomised controlled trials, as well as surveys. Chapter 7, *Analysing quantitative data and understanding basic statistics*, takes up some introductory ideas in quantitative research methods of data analysis. Chapter 8, *Using and critiquing systematic reviews and meta-analyses*, presents some details on how students can plan a protocol for a systematic review as well as introducing some basic concepts in this area for qualitative, quantitative and mixed methods reviews.

The last section is Section 4: *Writing and finishing*. This section will help you produce an acceptable finished product for your work. Chapter 9 is called *Writing up your literature review and documentary analysis*, and Chapter 10 looks at issues in *Writing your research proposal and dissertation*.

Concluding remarks are offered at the end of the book.

Learning features

The book is interactive. You are encouraged to work through it as an active participant, taking responsibility for your learning, in order to increase your knowledge, understanding and ability to apply this learning to practice.

Case studies throughout the book will help you to examine the theoretical material discussed in the context of nursing practice. We have devised activities that require you to reflect on experiences, situations and events and help you to review and summarise learning undertaken. In this way your knowledge will become deeply embedded as part of your development. When you come to applying your learning in practice the reflection undertaken here will help you to understand the relevance of research concepts to practice.

This book will introduce knowledge and learning activities for you as a student nurse concerning the central processes relating to research in all areas of the discipline. Suggestions for further reading are made at the end of each chapter.

Section 1
Getting started

Chapter 1
Getting started on your final-year project

Chapter aims

After reading this chapter, you should have developed an understanding of these areas:

- nursing and research;
- an overview of literature reviews, project plans and dissertations;
- key terms in research;
- an introduction to quantitative and qualitative research paradigms and mixed methods approaches;
- research designs from particular traditions (including action research, evaluation research, participatory and emancipatory research, case studies);
- research attitude.

Introduction

You are about to embark upon a process that is likely to change the way you think. You will gain tools for challenging your own thinking and the thinking of others and get a glimpse 'behind the scenes' at how knowledge is created. As a result, you are likely to experience more freedom than with any other part of the course for intensive study of a topic that interests you.

Historically, nursing has seen itself as a 'practical' subject and has drawn upon other disciplines to provide a research base to inform its interventions. Medicine, sociology, psychology and biology have been the disciplines that have been the most influential; all of these have relatively well-established research bases. As nursing has evolved as a discipline and is now in the process of becoming an all-graduate profession, there has been a shift towards developing nursing's own research base.

The use of evidence to inform professional nursing practice (as opposed to looking after people based on custom-and-practice or tradition) is now widely established as essential (Ellis, 2013). Thus developing an understanding of research and related concepts such as literature searching and ethics is an important part of the pre-registration nursing degree, usually occurring in the later course years. So you will have become accustomed to traditional academic writing and competence-based assessments such as placement portfolios; however, the prospect of learning a new vocabulary and set of skills can be a little daunting. For example, although all students must demonstrate numerical proficiency before qualifying, this may not translate into confidence in critically appraising statistical information. Even the language of research design, methodology and data analysis can seem technical and remote from students' experiences.

Activity 1.1   *Reflection*

Take a sheet of blank paper. Think of the term 'research' and jot down any ideas that occur to you.

Take a separate sheet of paper and jot down the emotions provoked by the idea of engaging in research.

As this is a personal reflective activity, there is no outline answer at the end of the chapter.

Some students find that a lot of negative emotions are forthcoming. Reinforcing negative emotions by going over them repeatedly will not help you to overcome them. It is very important that these are supplanted by some positives, so try the following: visualise yourself successfully completing your dissertation or module assignment, handing it in and getting a really good mark. How good would that feel? Next, think about how much you want to be a nurse – hopefully quite a lot at this stage of your programme. This is one module or assignment that is between you and your goal of becoming a nurse but it is achievable; thousands of students do something similar every year. Visualise yourself at your graduation, in your best clothes, with your friends and family clapping as you receive your certificate. Return to this imagery if things get tough when you are writing. You now have a positive goal in sight rather than negative emotions, and successfully completing your dissertation is just part of that.

For many nurses, 'research' is something that is either intimidating or boring – perhaps both. It is done by other people, such as psychologists or doctors, using highly complex and technical procedures. We hope to challenge these myths throughout this book and demonstrate to you that research is something that can be interesting and straightforward. For nurses, the point of research is not as a purely academic exercise but rather about how it contributes to improvements in everyday nursing practice and patient care. This is reflected in the Nursing and Midwifery Council (NMC) Standards for Pre-registration Nursing Education (NMC, 2010a) as well as their Essential Skills Clusters (NMC, 2010b) and the Quality Assurance Agency (QAA, 2001) subject benchmarks for nursing, listed in the Introduction. Whilst few nursing students will undertake a piece of research as a final-year project, many will be asked to undertake a *literature review*, often in conjunction with a research proposal. This book therefore focuses on these aspects: it is about understanding and doing literature reviews and applying research concepts to proposal writing, rather than about research *per se*.

The purpose of such extended pieces of work is that they provide an opportunity to explore and develop key, transferable academic skills such as project management, analysis and synthesis, and critiquing and developing a deeper understanding of research and evidence to underpin practice.

By reviewing the literature in an area, you will also gain indepth knowledge of a topic that you are interested in from the practice setting. As an overview, undertaking a literature review involves an exhaustive search and retrieval exercise using a systematic process of:

- searching electronic databases using key words;
- specifying criteria for the retrieval of articles from the search;
- using critical appraisal to examine the articles' strengths and weaknesses, usually against some agreed criteria;
- synthesis of the literature to uncover some insights (possibly new ones) as evidenced by this body of knowledge.

An important development in nursing and healthcare in this field is that of systematic reviews and meta-analyses. This usually applies to quantitative work, although there are qualitative, narrative approaches to it. We explore these concepts more fully in Chapter 8.

Writing a project proposal will be useful and you will gain from the experience because, as well as requiring you to understand research concepts more fully and plan a coherent study, it may inform future studies such as a Master's degree. You will also be addressing the professional standards listed in the Introduction and these in turn will influence your patient care when you are qualified.

Research project proposals need to include a summary of the literature on the topic you have chosen. This summary may or may not need to be sourced in a systematic review, but it will need to contain a background and rationale for the proposal and some idea about how the existing literature informs your study. You will need to have a research question, a sentence with a question mark at the end, as well as aims and objectives. Ensure that these are achievable and not too ambitious! You will probably be asked to write about your underlying approach, whether qualitative or quantitative. You would then develop an outline of how you intend to conduct the study, indicating what methods of data collection and analysis you will use (this is why we spend time below outlining some of the different ways in which this can be understood), as well as a timetable, resources and plan for dissemination of the findings.

'Dissertation' is a term that is applied to some form of extended study, usually undertaken as part of an academic award. For our purposes, it can denote a third-year piece of work, with an element of choice involved. Dissertations do not usually take an essay format, in which students are asked to answer a question; rather, they require students to choose an area of practice of their own interest and explore that in some way. A dissertation would normally have some element of research in it, and the term is most frequently associated with a research project where data collection and analysis are carried out, although this is not common in nursing courses. In nursing, a dissertation could be a project where literature is reviewed and conclusions and recommendations drawn, and may include a research proposal. You may not even have a 'dissertation module'; if you do have one, be careful to write following the structure requirements given at your institution. As it is usually worth more than the normal number of credits it is perhaps 5,000 words or longer, and will involve an element of critical appraisal, analysis and synthesis.

Transferable skills

Completing your project will provide you with the following range of transferable skills:

- project management skills, from first conception through to completion. These include time management and planning skills as well as evaluation and implementation skills;
- the ability to find and begin to critically evaluate research studies, rather than accepting them at face value. This can lead to increased confidence to question your own practice and the practice of others;
- the ability to think and study independently and take responsibility for your own learning as an autonomous practitioner. This can lead to increased curiosity and openness to new ideas.

These are all essential skills that will increase your employability and positively improve your practice.

Professional development and reflective practice

Great emphasis is placed on developing skills of reflection about, in and on practice. This has developed over many years in nursing. It is important also that you reflect on practice.

Developing a questioning approach that looks in a critical way at how you approach the research task and seeks to heighten your skills will help you to refine your practice and deepen your understanding of research concepts. Reflection is central to good nursing practice, but only if action results from that reflection.

Reflecting about, in and on your practice is not only important during your nurse preparation programme; it is considered key to continuing professional development. As we move to a profession that acknowledges lifelong learning as a way of keeping up to date, ensuring that research informs practice and honing skills and values for practice, it is important to begin the process at the outset of your development. This is reinforced by the NMC (2010a, b) and QAA (2001) standards discussed in the Introduction.

The role of research in your projects

We will now look over the key terms and approaches in research, some of which you may have come across before, to help you recall these prior to starting on your project. Although you may not be working with all these methods within your course, you will need to be familiar with them, and their application in nursing, in order to complete a research proposal or plan, and to assess literature as part of your literature review.

Future chapters will look at each of these in more detail to enable you to select the most appropriate methods for your research proposal. So consider the notes below as a 'refresher', which we will then go on to cover in more detail and relate more closely to study design. We have begun by asking you to reflect upon your initial thoughts about engaging in research. Below, you will be introduced to key terms. The distinction between quantitative and qualitative approaches will be discussed. You will be asked to consider a range of research designs from particular traditions to illustrate the wide diversity of approaches.

Key terms in research

As with any new area of study, you need to understand new terminology that can seem technical and confusing. Here are a few key terms that you will come across when studying for, and considering the design of, your research proposal or project. There is considerable debate about the exact use of specific terms, but the definitions below are generally agreed upon and are the meanings that are used in this book.

Data refers to the information that you are going to collect in order to answer your research question; for example, the words used by your interview participants or numerical information from your questionnaires. Strictly speaking, data is a plural rather than a singular noun (the singular is 'datum') and this convention will be kept throughout this book.

Epistemology is the study of knowledge and addresses the question of what counts as legitimate knowledge. Research projects contain assumptions about what is legitimate knowledge, and this is known as its *epistemological position* or *stance*.

Methodology refers to the totality of how you are going to undertake your research. It includes the research approach that you will use, including your epistemological position and the specific research methods you will choose, such as interviews or questionnaires.

Research approach or *paradigm* refers to the traditional division between quantitative and qualitative traditions in research, which will be discussed further in this chapter.

Research method refers to the practical way in which you are going to collect your data. Commonly used methods in healthcare research are interviews, questionnaires, *focus groups* and rating scales.

Sampling refers to the process of selecting the participants (or other data sources, e.g. documents) that will be involved in your study. Your *sample* (the selection of people or other data sources) is chosen from the total possible data sources, known as the *population*.

Research participants replaces the outmoded term 'research subjects', because the latter term suggests that people involved in research should have a passive role in a process to which they are 'subjected'. The term 'participants' suggests a more active and equal role, in which participation is informed and freely chosen.

Quantitative research tends to emphasise quantification and measurement, which can be analysed using statistical tests to establish a relationship between variables (e.g. poor mental health and social exclusion). Where there are testable hypotheses – which are predictions such as that higher levels of mental ill health are likely to be linked to higher levels of social exclusion – statistical tests can be used to establish relationships in these data.

Qualitative research tends to emphasise words as data, such as the words of participants in interviews or written data from documents. Rather than testing hypotheses, qualitative research seeks to explain the meaning of social phenomena through exploring the ways in which individuals understand their social worlds. More recently, data in visual forms such as photographs or films have been an increasingly popular subject of study.

Quantitative versus qualitative research

In its simplest formulation, quantitative research asks 'what is going on here?' or 'which option is better than the other?' Qualitative research, on the other hand, asks 'what is the meaning of what is happening?' For example, a quantitative study may measure the rates for mental ill health and social exclusion for a sample of mental health service users and find that there is a link (i.e. people with higher rates of mental ill health are likely to experience higher rates of social exclusion). A qualitative study would explore the meaning of what is happening, for example whether people with mental health problems are experiencing stigma and prejudice, whether participants are isolating themselves as a means of coping with distressing symptoms or some other explanation. Both approaches can provide useful insights into a particular research topic and there is a growing recognition of the strengths of mixed methodologies (Plano Clarke and Cresswell, 2008). Actually, neither approach is 'better' than the other; it is simply deciding which is more appropriate for the research question, and the question should come before the choice of methodology because the type of question asked determines how it will be investigated. When planning a research project or developing a proposal for a module or in a clinical setting, deciding on your research question leads you to choose a research approach which is best suited to answering it. Qualitative and quantitative research approaches are considered in more detail later in the book.

Quantitative research

Quantitative research tends to follow a traditional scientific model, which emphasises 'objectivity' by seeking to remove the values and attitudes of the researcher from the study. There is an emphasis on studying causal relationships and formulating fixed rules for the process of inquiry (Humphries, 2008). Sampling issues are particularly important because of the emphasis on being able to create statistical generalisations that are applicable to the wider population.

Quantitative research and positivism

Quantitative research has been influenced by *positivism* as an approach to knowledge. Every approach to research has underlying assumptions about the nature of knowledge and the social world, which is referred to as its *epistemological position* (see above, page 13). Positivism as an epistemological position traces its intellectual heritage back to Auguste Comte and argues that the traditional scientific method applied in the natural sciences is appropriate to the study of society (Giddens, 1993). From a positivist stance, the researcher is seen as an objective observer whose role is to infer laws that explain relationships between observed phenomena (Giddens, 2006).

Gray (2004) identifies three major claims of positivism:

1. Reality is viewed as consisting only of what can be experienced through the senses. Consequently, phenomena that cannot directly be sensed (e.g. people's intentions, wishes and fears) are not suitable as a subject for scientific inquiry.
2. Inquiry should be based upon scientific observations rather than philosophical speculation, and therefore on empirical inquiry.
3. The natural and human sciences are similar as they share common logical and methodological principles. This includes the belief that facts can be distinguished from values.

Although positivism dominated the social sciences for much of the twentieth century, it has fallen from favour since the 1980s as critics have challenged its core assumptions and its appropriateness for researching the complexities of our social world (Payne and Payne, 2004, page 171).

The challenges to positivism have led to a more sophisticated version of the traditional scientific approach known as realism, which is becoming increasingly influential. This is a broad range of approaches variously named as 'scientific realism', 'critical realism', 'subtle realism' and 'transcendental realism', each of which has a slightly different emphasis (Robson, 2011). An increasingly popular approach is critical realism (Bhaskar, 1978, 1979, 1990), which believes that there is an external reality but sees the concepts that we use to understand it as a provisional way of knowing rather than a direct reflection of reality. This approach also allows for theoretical content that is not amenable to direct observation, which would not be acceptable in positivism (Bryman, 2012).

You are likely to come across the randomised controlled trial (RCT) in your literature reviews, as this is a particularly influential research approach in healthcare and nursing, involving what is known as an experimental design. We will discuss experimental designs and RCTs briefly below (pages 21–23) and then further in Chapter 6, but in essence they are ways of assessing the effectiveness of different 'treatments' to find out which one works best relative to others. They are increasingly popular and reported in nursing journals for all branches and specialities in nursing, and are frequently described as the 'gold standard' in healthcare research.

Qualitative research

Qualitative research tends to use data in the form of words rather than numerical information. It seeks to explain social phenomena through understanding the ways in which individuals make sense of their social worlds and sees knowledge as historically and culturally situated (Crotty, 1998, page 67). In qualitative research, there are no clearly defined rules about sample size, but generally smaller sample sizes are used and studied in more depth and detail (Miles and Huberman, 1994). The primary focus is the importance of understanding individuals' own accounts of their perceptions, views and feelings and the meanings they attach to social phenomena.

Qualitative research and interpretivism

Qualitative research has been influenced by *interpretivism* as an epistemological position. Interpretivism is a broad term used to describe a range of approaches that challenge the traditional scientific approach of positivism. Interpretivism argues that the research methods of the natural sciences (from where positivism originated) are inappropriate to study social phenomena because they do not take into account the viewpoints of the social actors involved. For example, identifying the reasons for young people's unhealthy behaviour such as drug taking or unprotected sex requires the nurse researcher to understand the perspectives of the key social actors. The intellectual origins of interpretivism can be traced back to the nineteenth and early twentieth centuries as thinkers began to develop ways of researching, understanding and interpreting people's experiences of life (Bryman, 2012).

Quantitative research is generally more valued by governmental bodies as it focuses more on 'what works' and is more easily generalisable. Medical research uses this approach extensively whereas nursing research has tended to favour qualitative approaches. More recently, there has been a trend towards combining these methodologies, so traditional distinctions have become blurred.

Qualitative research and reflexivity

Whereas quantitative research seeks to remove the researcher from the study through addressing issues of bias, qualitative researchers argue that this is neither possible nor necessarily desirable. We bring our background and identity to our research, but from a traditional perspective this is viewed as a problem (a source of bias) rather than a valuable component of the research (Maxwell, 1996). In qualitative research, this is developed through the concept of *reflexivity*, which acknowledges that we bring our own thoughts, values and beliefs as well as our ethnicity, race, class, gender, sexual orientation, occupation, family background and schooling to our research (Kirby and McKenna, 1989).

Reflexivity has been defined as the *practice of researchers being self-aware of their own beliefs, values and attitudes, and their personal effects on the setting they have studied, and self-critical about their research methods and how they have been applied* (Payne and Payne, 2004, page 191). Reflexivity can ensure high standards because it involves the researcher constantly reviewing the process of investigation. Huberman and Miles (1998) argue for the researcher documenting the research process. This has been referred to as an 'audit trail', which explains why decisions were made (Lincoln and Guba, 1985) and should be regarded as a resource rather than a defensive action (Payne and Payne, 2004).

Feminist research has a long tradition of promoting qualitative research as an appropriate strategy for studying social phenomena in context. Feminist research is not so much a specific research design or method, but an approach to research that is informed by a set of values. These values recognise the power differentials that exist within wider society and within academic discourses, which have favoured patriarchal models of research that emphasise objectivity and distance between the researcher and the researched. It emphasises reflexivity as part of the rejection of these models, and as a resource for a radical paradigm shift (Payne and Payne, 2004). Feminist research tends to be antipositivist, although it includes quantitative as well as qualitative research methods. It places gender at the centre of social inquiry, investigating and representing the diversity of women's perspectives (Sarantakos, 2005).

Generic qualitative research

When undertaking research studies using the designs listed below under the heading 'Research designs from particular traditions', it is necessary to adhere to these designs quite scrupulously, or rigour can suffer. More recently, a trend amongst some qualitative researchers is for what has become known as 'generic qualitative research' (Caelli et al., 2003). This is an approach that uses methods of data collection from the qualitative tradition, without some of the other methodological assumptions that come with the traditional qualitative schools of thought.

So, in summary, qualitative research is an approach which seeks to understand people's experiences in particular situations. This is useful in nursing because it can give us insight into the issues involved in, for example, living with illnesses, or being a patient or client and using services, or being marginalised or disadvantaged in some way. With an enhanced understanding of these areas, nurses can begin to think through how they can alter their care and tailor their services more effectively to meet the needs of their patients and clients. Such studies are usually quite small-scale and based in a local context, so we can't automatically assume that the findings relate exactly to our own care settings, but qualitative work is often used where little is known about particular issues and it is a start (at least) to know things from small, local studies.

For those undertaking modules and planning projects, a research question seeking to understand or interpret people's experiences will lead to the use of a qualitative approach. This may be useful when little is known in an area of your own interest in practice, or as an attempt to evaluate issues in your own care setting, or relating to your own service delivery. We look in more detail at qualitative designs in Section 3.

Research designs from particular traditions

When planning your project or undertaking a literature review, you will need to be able to identify and understand a range of research designs from different traditions. What follows is a brief introduction to these which will help you gain an overview before starting your project. This is not exhaustive; neither is it intended as a menu from which you must choose. The aim is to illustrate the rich diversity in approaches to research design and the values that underpin them. The approaches are discussed in alphabetical order to challenge the idea that some designs are 'better' than others. To reiterate: the 'best' research design is the one that allows you to answer your research question!

We have suggested further reading for each of the designs covered below at the end of the chapter.

Action research and participatory action research

Action research challenges the traditional conception of the researcher as separate from the real world seeking theoretical knowledge that makes little difference in practice. It is associated with smaller-scale research projects that seek to address real-world problems, particularly amongst practitioners who want to improve practice, with a more equal and collaborative relationship between researchers and participants occurring as a feature of the study design. Rather than merely studying the social world, action research seeks to change it in practical ways. Another feature of action research is a view of the research process as being cyclical, in the sense that findings are fed back directly into practice in an ongoing process (Denscombe, 2007).

Action research traces its intellectual history to the work of Kurt Lewin, a social psychologist working in poor communities in post–Second World War America (Humphries, 2008). Action research is not a specific research method. It is more an approach to research that stresses the importance of links with real-world problems and a belief that research should serve practical ends. It is compatible with a wide range of research methods, ranging from experimental to phenomenological designs.

Participatory action research (*PAR*) is a form of action research that is committed to the involvement of those who are most affected (Alston and Bowles, 1998). It challenges the traditional power imbalance between the researcher as 'expert' and research participant as 'passive subject' and is highly compatible with antidiscriminatory and antioppressive practice, as the focus is to change participants' situations for the better under their direction.

There are also a number of similar approaches, such as 'appreciative inquiry' and 'cooperative inquiry'. These share a commitment to promoting the empowerment of participants, but each has a different emphasis (Heron and Reason, 2006; Ludema et al., 2006).

Koch et al. (2008) illustrate how a PAR study can be used to give voice to those who are usually marginalised as well as to illuminate practice issues and day-to-day changes. They studied how women with multiple sclerosis (MS) and urinary incontinence perceive the daily challenges they encounter. Four female MS sufferers, the researcher and two continence nurse advisers (CNAs) met on five occasions and the group interactions were recorded and transcribed. As well as finding four themes in the interactions (maintaining control; seeking understanding; avoiding shame; and good and bad days), the women and the CNAs were able to discuss living with MS and incontinence from their differing perspectives. The CNAs learned much about the women's experience and have changed their daily practice as a result.

These are fascinating and increasingly influential forms of research, but if you are choosing this for a method in your project plan, be aware that their innovative nature can make them problematic if they are not fully understood by students and supervisors, or if timescales are limited by the need to adhere to strict deadlines. Genuine participatory research requires considerable time to develop because the project's development is steered in the directions in which participants want to take it. This makes it difficult to predict at the outset where it will end up and how long it will take to achieve change; this uncertainty can involve ethical issues too (Williamson and Prosser, 2002).

Case studies

A *case study* is a detailed inquiry into a single example of a phenomenon, whether it is an organisation, individual, event, process, location or period of time (David, 2006). Rather than a research method, it is more a focus of study in which a variety of research methods can be used. These can range from experimental methods within a quantitative approach through to ethnography using observation and interviews within a qualitative approach. In practice, however, most case studies tend to adopt a qualitative approach (Payne and Payne, 2004) and are relatively descriptive.

Yin (2009) argues that case study research has traditionally been regarded as a 'weak sibling' compared to other research designs, such as experimental studies. This has changed in recent years as qualitative research has become more accepted within health and social sciences. A traditional criticism of case studies is whether findings can be generalised. For example, the statistical generalisations produced by large-scale statistical analysis would not be possible from a case study; this would be inappropriate because the case is studied in its own right rather than as an example of a particular class (Payne and Payne, 2004).

Yin (2009) identifies three types of case study. The *critical case* is chosen because it has features that challenge an existing theory or hypothesis. The *unique case* is chosen because its distinctiveness is its merit, although it may provide ways of understanding more usual cases. The *revelatory case* is chosen because it can provide new insights and ideas.

Courtenay et al. (2009) conducted a case study to explore issues in consultations between nurse prescribers and dermatology patients, as they wanted to illustrate the unique contribution of nurses to patient care. Ten practice settings were evaluated using a mixed methods approach, including questionnaires, interviews and videoed observations of consultations. The researchers found that nurses believed their holistic approach to assessment and prescribing improved prescribing decisions, while patients valued nurses' skills in listening and in explaining treatments.

If you were choosing a case study approach you would need to be clear that you were investigating some aspect of local practice or patients' experiences, and that your research and findings would be highly context-specific and not necessarily relevant elsewhere. This doesn't mean that you shouldn't conduct this type of research: it may be very useful and desirable that local service delivery or patients' experiences are evaluated and the findings shared more widely. These comments also apply to the discussion of evaluation research, below.

Clinical data mining

Clinical data mining (CDM) is a practice-based research strategy for systemically collecting and analysing available agency data such as medical, nursing, allied health and other hospital records (Epstein, 2009). CDM offers a promising and practical research approach for academics, but is particularly attractive to research-minded practitioners and postgraduate degree students. For example, it can be used by practitioners to evaluate their own interventions and reflect upon their own practice. It is generally used retrospectively to analyse existing data but could be combined with original data collection. Likewise, it can provide data for Master's and PhD degree studies on topics difficult to study via original data collection.

Epstein (2009) describes three basic types of CDM studies. The first type directly converts existing quantitative data to a quantitative database for statistical analysis. The second type converts data that were originally in narrative form (e.g. nursing notes) from qualitative form to a quantitative database for statistical analysis. The third type is purely qualitative data, where narrative data receive a qualitative analysis.

Case study

Patients with life-threatening liver disease go through a two-stage process at the Mount Sinai Medical Center in New York City to determine their eligibility for transplants. After they are determined as medically appropriate for transplant, patients then have a second assessment to determine their suitability for a transplant on psychosocial grounds. Since the shortage of donor organs means that only about half of requests can be accepted, the psychosocial assessment is crucial for patients. Staff team members and a research consultant extracted quantitative data about psychosocial risk factors and outcomes from around 500 former patients in order to complete the largest retrospective study of patient psychosocial risk factors and liver transplant mortality ever completed in the transplant literature (Epstein et al., 1997).

CDM has a number of strengths. First, it is practitioner-friendly and it explicitly promotes practitioners as researchers. Second, it is less resource-intensive than most other forms of research. Since the data are already available, the costly and time-consuming process of data collection is avoided, although data will usually need work to convert them into a suitable format. Third, it makes use of valuable data that already exist but which are rarely used for research purposes. Since the amount of data that is collected for research purposes is only a tiny fraction of the amount of data routinely collected for clinical purposes, the potential for knowledge creation is considerable. Finally, CDM is unobtrusive and more ethically sound than most other data-gathering approaches. It does not involve the patient risks or burdens involved in data collection (e.g. interviewing patients, relatives or staff about sensitive topics), nor does it involve the ethical risks involved in experimental or quasi-experimental studies (see below for more detailed discussion). The main limitation of CDM is that any research method that relies on clinical records is only as good as the available data sources themselves. Consequently, missing data, reliability questions and absent variables must be anticipated. However, once recognised, these issues can be minimised with proper safeguards.

Evaluation research

Evaluation research has become popular within healthcare as part of the drive for increased accountability of public services and the evidence-based practice agenda. Indeed, it is usually valued highly by practitioners, particularly when deciding between different interventions, allocating scarce resources or demonstrating that in-service innovations are effective.

To evaluate something is to assess its merits or worth. By definition, it cannot be value-neutral because there must be aims and standards against which something is judged (Humphries,

2008, page 170). In real life, evaluation is also rarely value-neutral in the sense that it can be used for organisational purposes. For example, evaluations can be used to justify closing a service or to promote the wider organisation.

Evaluation research requires you to develop specific criteria, which can be an interesting and fraught process as different stakeholders can have different perspectives. Senior management may be interested in cost-effectiveness and adherence to national standards and National Institute for Health and Care Excellence (NICE) guidelines, while service users may be more interested in how responsive the service is to their needs. There are obvious similarities with action research. However, one common difference is the role of the researcher. Whilst the researcher in action research is often in a practitioner role, this is less acceptable within evaluation research because it would be viewed as compromising objectivity.

Another related criticism of evaluation is that it is atheoretical in its approach; that is, it does not use wider theory drawn from the social sciences to inform its design. In many contexts, this is not problematic and studies do not need to demonstrate engagement with the wider academic literature in order to be effective and useful, providing that methods of data collection and analysis are rigorous. A final note of caution is that evaluation research can be politically sensitive, which can pose challenges for access and for researchers' relationships with service users and staff.

Service evaluations may utilise existing data and are similar in that respect to audit, or they may collect new data for a specific purpose. For example, Williamson et al. (2007) discuss a patient satisfaction survey of a nurse-led clinic for cancer care follow-up. Data were collected using a questionnaire, which evaluated the initial months of the clinic's existence. It was a new service and the nurse specialist and medical consultant wanted to understand the issues for patients and gain some perspective concerning what worked well, what might need to be altered, and what patients thought of the new service compared to the old medical-led arrangements. Overall, patients were satisfied with many aspects of the new service. While this service evaluation is highly context-specific, it illustrates how service redesign can take place as a result of national policy and clinical guidance, which had driven the changes. So, while Williamson et al.'s (2007) study evaluated satisfaction with the new service, they also generated some more widely applicable knowledge of relevance to similar services elsewhere or for the service user group as a whole.

Service evaluation is an important and growing area of healthcare research. Choosing a service evaluation as a project or for a proposal will allow you to gain skills in this area which may come in useful at a later stage in your career when you have more responsibility for service delivery. It may suit you that you will not need to adopt a theoretical position (such as grounded theory or phenomenology) if the aim of your research is to produce useable findings for understanding and improving patient care.

Experimental and quasi-experimental designs

These designs are similar to a traditional scientific approach and are most often used to evaluate interventions and test theories (known as *hypotheses*). It is sometimes stated that an experimental design is the most rigorous form of research, which is somewhat misleading as all forms of research can possess rigour. It is more accurate to say that this is the approach that places most emphasis on removing possible sources of bias, which is achieved through introducing a degree of randomisation at different stages of the process, and by 'blinding' participants and staff to which intervention is being offered (known as 'double blinding') where possible.

The classic experimental design is the *randomised controlled trial* (RCT), mentioned earlier (page 15), in which participants are randomly assigned to one of two groups: an experimental and a control group. The experimental group receives the intervention, whereas the control group does not, and the effects are then measured in each group. Having a control group receiving no intervention raises ethical issues, because it requires one group not to receive a potentially beneficial intervention. This is less ethically problematic when there is little evidence as yet that the intervention is effective, but becomes more so as there is evidence that participants would be likely to benefit, and so a new treatment could be compared to an existing one. So, for example, if researchers wanted to answer the question, 'What is the best treatment for high blood pressure?' they would investigate this by giving one medication to one group of patients and comparing the outcomes with another drug given to another group of similar patients. Statistical tests would be used to establish the importance of these outcomes and whether or not they could be generalised to a wider population from the sample in which they were observed.

RCTs form one end of a spectrum of experimental and quasi-experimental approaches that can be used. We discuss the distinctions between experimental and quasi-experimental designs more fully in Section 3: briefly, a full experimental design would contain more rigorous features than a quasi-experimental design such as double blinding (where neither researcher nor patients would know which new treatment was given to avoid any subliminal biases being introduced), or a control group who were receiving no treatment or an existing one for the purposes of comparison. A common quasi-experimental design is a pre- and post-test design, in which one group of participants experiences an intervention and key variables are measured before and after the intervention to establish whether there has been a change.

For example, Chiang and Sun (2009) investigated whether introducing a walking programme for Chinese Americans would reduce their hypertension (high blood pressure) rates, with one group experiencing the programme, and another experiencing a culturally modified programme (aimed at being attractive to them as older Chinese Americans). There were no significant effects upon participant blood pressure or walking endurance as a result of either programme, and the study indicated that the walking protocol is appropriate to use without additional cultural modification.

This study illustrates how a quasi-experimental design might be useful in investigating variables which cannot rigorously be controlled or blinded: it was not possible to blind researchers and participants to allocated groups as patients were receiving different input from researchers and behaving differently as a result. This was obvious to the researchers, meaning that the full experimental control associated with a true experimental design is not present in this study. If you are thinking about constructing an experimental design, it is worth noting that the full features (which we discuss in Section 3) do not need to be present, and although quasi-experimental designs are not as robust as fully experimental ones, they can be used successfully.

Narrative approaches

There has been increasing interest in narrative approaches across the social sciences (Squire et al., 2008; Gubrium and Holstein, 2009). Narrative approaches are interested in the *storied nature of human conduct* (Sarbin, 1986), in which we respond to experiences by constructing stories and listening to the stories of others.

Narratives have been provisionally defined as *discourses with a clear sequential order that connects events in a meaningful way for a definite audience and thus offer insights about the world* (Hinchman and Hinchman, 1997, page xvi). However, such definitions are in dispute and the process of analysis does not offer the tightly prescribed procedures prevalent in approaches such as *grounded theory* (Riessman, 1993, 2007; Andrews et al., 2008).

Elliott (2005, page 6) identifies the following common themes in narrative research:

- an interest in people's lived experiences and an appreciation of the temporal nature of that experience;
- a desire to empower research participants and allow them to contribute to determining the most salient themes in the area of research;
- an interest in process and change over time;
- an interest in the self and representations of the self;
- an awareness that the researcher him- or herself is also a narrator.

Narrative research is often interested in issues of identity as stories play a central role in the formation of identity (Crossley, 2007, page 135). Indeed, Mair asserts that:

> *Stories are the womb of personhood. Stories make and break us. Stories sustain us in times of trouble and encourage us towards ends that we would not otherwise envision.*
> (Mair, 1989, page 2)

The history of narrative approaches to research can be traced back to two different academic traditions (Rustin, 2000; Andrews et al., 2004; Squire et al., 2008). The first is the post–Second World War rise of humanistic approaches within psychology and sociology as a reaction against positivism. The second is the influence within the humanities of a range of developments from Russian structuralist, French poststructuralist, postmodern, psychoanalytic and deconstructionist approaches to narrative (Squire et al., 2008).

There is a range of approaches to narrative research and a commonly made distinction is between event-centred and experience-centred approaches. Event-centred approaches focus upon *the spoken recounting of particular past events that happened to the narrator* (Squire et al., 2008, page 5) and are influenced by the work of Labov (Labov and Waletsky, 1967). Experience-centred approaches have a broader focus and explore stories that *may be about general or imagined phenomena, things that happened to the narrator or distant matters that they've only heard about* and can include writing and visual materials as well as speech (Squire et al., 2008, page 5).

The interest in people's lived experiences and in questions of identity mean that narrative research is particularly appropriate for understanding the experiences of trauma and researching sensitive issues (Crossley, 2000, 2007). Examples of narrative research include an autobiographical study of cancer (Frank, 1995), a study of men living with a long-term HIV diagnosis (Davies, 1997) and a historical study of how mental health service users' 'voices' have changed over time (Crossley and Crossley, 2001).

If you were going to choose a narrative approach for your own study or proposal, this could be a good way of giving voice to people who are not usually heard and to engage in a long dialogue with many people, particularly if the potential of electronic communications such as e-mail is utilised sensitively and effectively to interact with participants (Kralik et al., 2006).

A research attitude

Whichever research approach and design are chosen, it is important for you as a researcher to develop a 'research attitude'. This is about being rigorous in your thinking and willing to challenge yourself and others in a responsible way. This has been expressed by Robson (2011) as follows:

- Being systematic: giving serious thought to what is being done and how and why it is being done. This involves considering alternatives and making an argument for the choices made.
- Being sceptical: subjecting ideas to scrutiny and possible disconfirmation. This involves researchers asking themselves what evidence exists for the points they are making and considering alternative explanations.
- Being ethical: working within acceptable parameters. This involves following ethical frameworks, particularly those of the NHS Research Ethics Service and the NHS Trust research governance processes, as well as thinking about how their research might affect others (Robson, 2011, page 18), the potential clinical significance of their work and the need to comply with the requirements of professional bodies such as the NMC (Williamson, 2001).

Chapter summary

This chapter has asked you to reflect upon your initial thoughts about engaging in research. You have been introduced to key terms in research, and the distinction between quantitative and qualitative approaches to research was discussed. You have been asked to consider a range of research designs from particular traditions to illustrate the wide diversity of approaches.

In the next chapter we will look at how to undertake a literature review, and appraise and use research to inform practice.

Further reading

General

Bryman, A (2012) *Social Research Methods*, 4th edition. Oxford: Oxford University Press.
An excellent, all-round textbook that covers all aspects of the research process, including chapters on different methods (such as experimental and non-experimental methods).

Ellis, P (2013) *Evidence-Based Practice in Nursing*, 2nd edition. London: Sage/Learning Matters.
Clear and simple book which helps develop skills in the identification, appraisal and application of evidence for nursing practice.

Kvale, S and Brinkmann, S (2008) *InterViews: Learning the Craft of Qualitative Research Interviewing*, 2nd edition. London: Sage.
Second edition of a classic text firmly within the qualitative approach, which provides an interesting and detailed account of the differences between positivist and interpretative approaches.

Parahoo, K (2006) *Nursing Research: Principles, Process and Issues*, 2nd edition. Basingstoke: Palgrave Macmillan.
Comprehensive research methods text.

Action research and participatory action research

Coghlan, D and Brannick, T (2010) *Doing Action Research in Your Own Organisation*, 3rd edition. London: Sage.
Really good text which deals succinctly with key issues, including methodology and implementation.

Reason, P and Bradbury, H (eds) (2008) *Handbook of Action Research*, 2nd edition. London: Sage.
A useful collection of chapters by key figures in action research.

Williamson, G R, Bellman, L and Webster, J (2012) *Action Research in Nursing and Healthcare*. London: Sage.
This is an excellent resource for nurses and other healthcare professionals seeking to understand and use action research in their clinical practice.

Case studies

Yin, R (2008) *Case Study Research: Design and Methods*, 4th edition. London: Sage.
The classic text on case study design.

Clinical data mining

Epstein, I (2010) *Clinical Data-Mining: Integrating Practice and Research*. New York: Oxford University Press.
An excellent and interesting account of a new approach to documentary analysis. An insightful and entertaining read.

Evaluation research

Hall, I and Hall, D (2004) *Evaluation and Social Research: Introducing Small-Scale Practice*. Basingstoke: Palgrave Macmillan.
A useful guide that presents practical advice and real-life examples.

Pawson, R and Tilley, N (1997) *Realistic Evaluation*. London: Sage.
A classic and provocative text from the realist tradition.

Experimental and quasi-experimental designs

Bryman, A (2012) Research designs, in *Social Research Methods*, 4th edition. Oxford: Oxford University Press.
An excellent resource for students using social science research methods.

Parahoo, K (2006) Experiments, in *Nursing Research: Principles, Process and Issues*, 2nd edition. Basingstoke: Palgrave Macmillan.
One of the seminal research methods texts for nurses.

Narrative approaches

Andrews, M, Squire, C and Tamboukou, M (eds) (2008) *Doing Narrative Research*. London: Sage.
An excellent introduction to both the theoretical and practical dimensions of narrative research.

Riessman, C (2007) *Narrative Methods for the Human Sciences*. London: Sage.
An updated version of her classic 1993 text.

Useful websites

Organisations conducting and using research

http://wrap.warwick.ac.uk/230
The Centre for Evidence in Ethnicity, Health and Diversity.

www.jrf.org.uk
The Joseph Rowntree Foundation. Independent research foundation with useful publications on many subjects, including health and healthcare, poverty and social exclusion.

www.kingsfund.org.uk
The King's Fund. An independent charity seeking to improve healthcare. See their publication.

www.nice.org.uk
The National Institute for Health and Care Excellence. Provides clinical guidance on healthcare issues.

www.nihr.ac.uk
The National Institute for Health Research. Commissions and funds NHS and social care research and develops research evidence to support decision making by professionals.

www.rcn.org.uk/development/researchanddevelopment
The Royal College of Nursing Research and Development Co-ordinating Centre. Facilitates rather than conducts research but aims to increase the capacity of nurses working in research.

www.wellcome.ac.uk
The Wellcome Trust. Charity which funds medical and humanities research.

Research methods sources

www.methodspace.com
Methodspace. Research Methods' community resources and blog. By Sage Publishing.

www.oup.com/uk/orc/bin/9780199202959
Oxford University Press website. Online resources to support Bryman (2012).

www.socialresearchmethods.net
Web centre for social research methods. Collection of online resources for researchers.

Section 2
Planning and preparing for your final-year project

Chapter 2
Planning and undertaking a literature review or documentary analysis

Chapter aims

After reading this chapter, you should be able to:

- understand what a literature review is;
- feel confident about undertaking a literature search;
- understand what a documentary analysis is;
- feel confident about undertaking a documentary analysis;
- be able to source high-quality material in your topic area.

Introduction

You will have had some thoughts about your research topic and be starting to formulate your research question. The next stage is to undertake a literature review in order to establish what is already known about your research topics, and we will begin with this. We will then discuss documentary analysis, which is quite different from a literature review because it is a form of primary research in its own right. This chapter aims to guide you through that process, using case studies and activities to illustrate the different stages. This is a distinct process from conducting a systematic review and meta-analysis, which is a literature review undertaken using a strict, explicit and transparent set of formal protocols that seek to minimise the chances of systematic bias and error (Macdonald, 2003). We devote Chapter 8 to an introduction to systematic reviews and meta-analyses.

It is important to see your literature review as an ongoing process that would start in the early stages of planning your proposal, and would continue throughout the life of your project, if you were actually undertaking one. This would not be just about updating your literature review as new material becomes available: if you were undertaking data collection, these data would be likely to suggest new ways of looking at your research topic. Consequently, developing your literature review would be a continual process, in which you re-engaged with the literature as your project developed.

This chapter will begin by defining what is meant by a literature review and exploring its roles and functions. The process of undertaking a *literature search* will be reviewed, focusing on the challenge of finding high-quality material in your topic area. Chapter 9 looks at how a literature review and documentary analysis can be written up.

The procedures for undertaking a literature search and making effective notes will be examined. You will be asked to consider what it means to analyse critically the literature that you find and clear guidelines will be discussed. The process of writing up your literature review will be considered and some of the problems frequently encountered by students will be examined.

What is a literature review?

A literature review is a comprehensive summary and critical appraisal of the literature that is relevant to your research topic. It presents the reader with what is already known in this field and identifies traditional and current controversies as well as weaknesses and gaps in the field.

The terms *literature search* and *literature review* are sometimes treated as if they were synonymous, but a literature search refers to a systematic process of identifying material that is appropriate whereas a literature review refers to a critical evaluation of that material.

In a traditional dissertation (or a research article), you will discuss what you found in the body of literature at two stages. First, you will present it in your literature review to demonstrate your understanding of what has already been written in your field. This will be used to inform your study design. You then revisit it after your findings to discuss any similarities and differences between what you found and what previous researchers have found. In a proposal, you will only use the literature to create an introductory argument or give background to the study, which will also inform the study design.

Hart (2001) identifies two key areas when you begin a research project or write a proposal: the literature relevant to your research topic and the literature on research *methodology* (i.e. how to plan and conduct research). This is an important distinction because you are likely to have only searched for the former during your previous academic study. Reading this book is an excellent start to developing your knowledge of the latter and each chapter contains recommended texts for further reading.

There are many reasons for undertaking a literature review. It is an essential part of your project planning (and would form a necessary part of any project you might actually undertake). A systematic review and meta-analysis might also be acceptable for Master's qualification instead of an empirical research project (i.e. where you collect your own data), and might form part of a dissertation or extended study project in third-year undergraduate nursing programmes. It enables you to gain an understanding of what has already been written about your topic, including reviewing which research designs have been used and the key issues that have been identified. Consequently, it is an essential part of developing expertise in your field, both in the topic area and in research methodology, and will inform your project plan.

Conducting your literature search

A literature search is the first stage in your literature review and is an organised investigation for material relevant to your topic across a range of sources. In your previous studies, you may have concentrated on using textbooks to inform your coursework. The purpose of textbooks is to provide students with an overview of what is generally agreed in a particular field. Although textbooks may report the results of research studies, they may not be sufficiently current or detailed for the purposes of your literature review. You need to expand the range of literature that you utilise and this should include reading the original research studies themselves to be able to appraise them critically.

Types of literature

The main types of literature that will be relevant are described below.

Journal articles in printed and electronic form

These are generally regarded as being of the highest quality because most journals are peer-reviewed. This means that articles submitted to the journals will be anonymised and sent out to reviewers with expertise in the field. These reviewers will evaluate the potential article and will submit detailed feedback that the author must address before it is of a publishable standard. This does not guarantee that everything in an article is correct, but it is relatively stringent. Whilst articles from non-refereed journals may be of a similar standard, they have not been through this process. Journals will state that they are peer-reviewed if this is the case and many search engines allow you to search for refereed journals only.

Books in printed and electronic form

There are good-quality control mechanisms built into book publishing, but they are not regarded as being as stringent as for peer-reviewed journals. You may be used to reading textbooks that provide you with a good overview of an area, but the research studies that they describe are likely to be classic studies rather than the most recent material.

Official and legal publications

These include legislation, policy and discussion documents as well as research studies and summaries of research findings in specific subject areas, such as hospital discharge or child protection. As well as governmental bodies, this includes material from other public organisations (e.g. Joseph Rowntree Foundation, NSPCC).

Systematic reviews and meta-analysis, clinical guidelines, National Service Frameworks

Systematic reviews and *meta-analyses* are exceptionally influential in medical, nursing and health-care research as they inform decision making and treatment options on a daily basis, and provide an evidence base for the national recommendations for standards of treatment and care produced by the National Institute of Health and Care Excellence (NICE) and other bodies, such as the Scottish Intercollegiate Guidelines Network (SIGN). The most important and influential body funding systematic reviews and meta-analyses is the Cochrane Collaboration, but such reviews are also often published in journals.

Clinical guidelines can be extremely authoritative if published by influential bodies such as NICE and SIGN, and have gone through extensive processes of literature search and review before conclusions relating to effectiveness and cost-effectiveness of new treatments are given. Many NHS Trusts develop their own guidelines, which go through clinical governance approval, but that does not necessarily mean that they are completely authoritative. National Service Frameworks (NSFs) also contain authoritative reviews of evidence and are important in signposting standards of care for particular groups. For example, the NSF for Older People (Department of Health, 2001) contains 369 references, weighted so that greater importance is given to systematic reviews and meta-analyses than expert opinion, and this contributes a great deal to the overall recommendations produced.

Grey literature

This is material that is not published through traditional commercial sources but is available through specialised sources (e.g. research reports from local public or voluntary organisations). It is often unclear what quality control systems have been used, but they may contain some very useful and relevant information. University libraries will have copies of PhD and MSc theses submitted at their institutions, and conference abstracts may be useful in identifying 'cutting-edge' work. Whether to include them in your literature review depends upon what other material you have found. If you have found similar material from more conventional sources, you may not need to include them. But such material can be very valuable as long as you recognise the relative authority and its strengths and weaknesses.

How do I start my literature search?

The focal point of your literature search will be a systematic examination of a number of electronic bibliographic databases, which will enable you to search effectively across a large number of journals. These are available through your university library and are often available to access remotely through your home computer.

Most databases have 'basic' and 'advanced' search engines, so try using the latter for more specific and detailed searches and combine your key words to find more relevant results. When you search using an electronic database, you will be provided with an abstract that summarises the study. If your university has a subscription to that journal, you will also be able to get access to the full text version. The content of most electronic databases consists of journal articles, but some may include references to other material, such as books, reports and websites. Since no bibliographic database contains every journal available, you will need to search a number of databases to ensure that you identify all of the material available. Google Scholar is also useful and recommended, although it is likely to throw up thousands of hits, of which only a few will be relevant. You should also search the Cochrane Collaboration website and the NHS Evidence website.

It is tempting to start searching immediately, but you should first put together a search profile. This will direct your search and should consist of the following:

- Your research question: this guides every aspect of your project. For example: 'What are the reasons for delays in hospital discharge for older people?' Make sure you express the research question as a full sentence with a question mark at the end.

- Key words: these are the main terms that relate to your research question, which you will use as search terms. They should include alternative terms that may be used in the literature; for example, using 'older people' but also alternative (and often out-of-date) terms such as 'elderly' or 'geriatric'.
- Parameters: these are any restrictions that will narrow down your search, such as a particular time period or country of research or factors related to the population studied (e.g. age, gender and ethnicity); for example, deciding that you want literature on hospital discharge delay from the UK and relating to older people rather than other age groups.
- PICO: The mnemonic PICO (Sackett et al., 1997) is a useful means of structuring a search. PICO stands for:

  o population (or illness or condition);
  o intervention (treatment or service);
  o control (or comparison);
  o outcome.

- Using PICO to write down for yourself exactly what you are searching for allows you to structure your search very clearly and make sure you don't go off track. You will always have a population (or illness or condition) in your search; you may not always have an intervention in the sense of a treatment option but this could also relate to service delivery; you may not have a control (comparison) unless experimental designs are involved and the outcomes may not be clearly articulated at the search stage. Even so, PICO can help plan your literature search. Another useful mnemonic is SPIDER (Cooke et al., 2012). This stands for:

  o sample;
  o phenomenon of interest;
  o design;
  o evaluation;
  o research type.

Case study: Developing key words

Joan decided that the research question that she is most interested in discovering literature on is identifying best practice in diabetic foot care. For her literature search, her first task is to develop a list of key words that she is going to use.

Activity 2.1   *Critical thinking*

What will Joan include in her search profile? What will she include in her research question, key words and parameters? What will she include in her PICO assessment?

There is a brief summary of answers at the end of the chapter.

It can be confusing and frustrating at first to use some electronic search engines because they use *Boolean operators.* This sounds technical, but it is a relatively simple system to enable you to narrow your search and find the most relevant resources. These are built into the advanced search functions and it is worth understanding how they work. Although each database uses them in slightly different ways, the general principles apply.

The three most commonly used Boolean operators are 'AND', 'OR' and 'NOT'. If you insert the word 'AND' between search terms (e.g. 'elderly' AND 'discharge') you will narrow your search to texts that contain both terms. If you insert the term OR between search terms, you will broaden your search to include texts that contain either term. These can usefully be combined; for example, 'elderly AND discharge OR hospital' will identify resources that discuss the elderly in the context of either discharge or hospital settings. If you insert the term 'NOT' this will exclude any resources containing the second search term. This is useful when it has more than one meaning and you wish to restrict it. For example, if your search term is 'counselling' and you want to exclude careers counselling, you would use 'counselling NOT careers counselling'. Another useful function is the truncation symbol (* ! #), which lets you type in the first part of a word and then the search engine will find alternative endings; for example, adolesc* will find adolescent, adolescents, adolescence, and so on.

It is important to be systematic about your searches to ensure that you have identified all the relevant literature. Having all of your material in one place means that you will not have to search through different notebooks or diaries to find a reference. This should include all the searches that you undertake, including the date, bibliographic database and search terms used. A popular format is an electronic word-processing document with dated entries that enable you to track the progress of your research and to search for specific words. If you prefer to work on physical copies, consider having a folder of A4 sheets that can be taken out and placed into a ring binder as you go along. Whichever format you choose, you should maintain regular electronic or photocopied back-ups to ensure that the material is not lost.

Make a record of when you undertake a search, including the key words you used and date. You will need to use more than one database because every database has a limited coverage. More importantly, make a references list as you go along so that you avoid having to search for a reference at the last minute. There are a number of reference manager software packages, such as Mendeley, EndNote, ProCite and RefWorks; these will allow you to get the citation style exactly correct. Your university is likely to have adopted one and it is worth becoming familiar with it because it will create a central database of references that can be adapted into different citation systems, meaning, for example, that if you were planning to publish your work in an article, you could automatically adjust all the references to the style of that journal if it was different from that used by your university. Some software, such as Mendeley, allows you to store your articles in PDF format ('portable document format': articles which look exactly as if you have printed them from a journal) and can automatically input details of the articles, though it is important to check these for accuracy.

An additional search method that can be productive (but far less systematic) is to review the references section of material that you have already obtained. This can be particularly helpful when you have found an article that directly responds to your research question, because the references section is likely to include relevant material. As you gather more articles and books, you may find the same texts being referred to. This usually indicates that these are central texts for your topic and should be included in your literature review. This form of searching can be quite fruitful, but rather haphazard and biased because the writers may not be familiar with all of the literature and may not have included material that they want to distance themselves from. Hence, it should be regarded as a supplement rather than a replacement for a full literature search using electronic databases. You can try this trick with authors' names, so you search for everything that a particular author has written, then try the same thing with all the co-authors on their papers. You can usually do this in the electronic databases you'll be using by clicking on the relevant buttons. Although not systematic, it does give you a feel for who is publishing what in a particular field.

Effective reading and note taking

Having identified suitable material, it is important that you are able to use effective reading and note-taking skills to make the most of the time that you have. Rather than printing everything and working your way through a large pile of material, use active reading skills to identify which material is most relevant and take appropriate notes. As you should be able to get electronic full-text PDFs, often it is not necessary to print the articles you find on paper if you are comfortable reading them on screen.

A classic technique (Robinson, 1970) for achieving this is known as the SQ3R reading strategy, which comprises the following five stages:

1. Survey (or skim): conduct a preliminary scan of the material to get a general sense of what the material is about. This may simply consist of reading the abstract if it is a journal article. Does it look relevant? If not, discard at this stage.
2. Question: actively ask yourself what the article or chapter is about and what questions it might answer in order to decide whether the text is worth reading more carefully.
3. Read the text more carefully if it has passed the above tests. Read actively, questioning the author's arguments, and make appropriate notes.
4. Recall (or recite) the main points when you have finished reading, using your own words.
5. Review: test yourself to see what you can recall. If there are sections that you cannot remember, you may need to reread the material.

One of the most useful tips for saving time and reducing stress is to make sure that you keep a note of the full reference for the material that you are reading. While this may seem like a nuisance at the time, it will be preferable to hunting around for it at the last minute, long after you originally read it. It is particularly important to keep the reference list of your proposal or project report up to date as you go along (unless you are using a reference manager software package such as Mendeley or EndNote, which will help you).

When you are reading and taking notes, try to make links with other material that you have read. When you read your first article, it is difficult to have a framework to judge it against. When you have read a number of articles, you will have a greater understanding of the literature and will find it easier to evaluate a particular article or book.

Case study: Recording searches

Susan developed a system for recording her literature searches and the material that she found. Using her research journal she recorded every search. She also noted the numbers of search hits and how she reduced large numbers of hits to those of more relevance to her interests, as these details are frequently needed in assignments and proposals, so that it can be shown that a search is systematic and inclusive rather than biased in some way.

Susan read the abstract of every article in order to gain a sense of what it contained. She decided to use a traffic light system to organise the material into three groups (red, amber and green lights). For some articles, reading the abstract was enough for her to realise that the article was not relevant to her research and was discarded at that stage (red light). Other articles looked very promising and highly relevant to her research topic so were grouped together (green light). A third group were articles that were potentially relevant, depending upon how her research developed (amber light). She decided to devote most of her attention to the 'green light' group in order to develop a good knowledge of her specific research topic but to keep material from the 'amber light' group in case her research changed as it developed.

If, like Susan, you used a traffic light system, you could mark all the printed papers and keep them together in a folder, or you could simply keep the PDFs in separate folders in your computer's memory. Using Endnote will allow you to catalogue very efficiently and insert citations directly into the text and reference list.

What if I find too much or too little material?

In literature searching it is highly unusual to get exactly what you want, in the quantity that you want it, first time around. Usually you will need to repeat searches in different databases, refine your search terms and search again and again. As you start your literature search, you may find yourself confronted with either too much or too little material. It is more common to find that your literature search has identified too much material. The development of digital technology has seen a revolution in the information that is available for your research compared to 10 or 15 years ago. The disadvantage of this is that it is easy to become overwhelmed by the sheer volume of information that is available. If you have identified too much material, your search is too broad and needs to be narrowed down. This can be done in a number of ways. First, you could be more specific about your topic. Second, you can be more specific about your parameters (e.g. choosing a specific time period or restricting your search to UK materials).

If you have identified too little material, you need to think about your search terms. Whereas some areas really do have very little written about them, it is more likely that your search terms are not finetuned enough to pick them up. If you have identified a small amount of material, read it to find out the terminology that is used in your research field. Think of alternative terms and enlist the help of your supervisor and/or fellow students in this task. If you still cannot identify any literature in your research field, it may be necessary to consider adjusting your research topic to ensure you have sufficient material to discuss in your literature review. If you genuinely cannot find anything on a subject area you will need to look at related subject areas for justification, rationale and methodological ideas concerning how you write your proposal.

Critically analysing the literature

In order to be worth including in your literature search, a text needs to be both relevant and of sufficient quality. Avoid the pitfall of reading material that is interesting, but not directly relevant to your research. This can take up a considerable amount of your time and the material is unlikely to feature in your final dissertation.

When you are evaluating a research study, there are a number of questions that you should ask yourself:

- Research design: does the study provide a clear rationale for the choice of research design? Research questions can usually be approached using a variety of research designs so a good study will provide a clear and robust rationale for its choices, including a discussion of why it did not use alternative designs.
- Data collection methods: does the study provide a clear rationale for the choice of data collection methods? For example, a study may have chosen interviews rather than questionnaires or focus groups. Is a coherent account given for this choice? Were known weaknesses addressed and did the data collection methods work in practice?
- Sampling: how well do the sampling procedures match the research question? Sampling is particularly important in quantitative research because this limits the extent to which the findings can be generalised. Were known weaknesses addressed and did the sampling procedures work in practice?
- Data analysis: how robust is the data analysis? A good study will give a clear account of how the data were analysed, whether quantitative or qualitative. Does the data analysis follow the model described? If it is a quantitative study using statistical analysis, are the tests used appropriate? Please see the end of the chapter for recommended texts on quantitative data analysis and www.socialresearchmethods.net to provide a useful guide to appropriate statistical tests. If it is a qualitative study, does the analysis provide sufficient context for the material to be understandable? Does it account for the diversity of participants' views?
- Credibility of the findings: how credible are the findings? You need to consider whether the conclusions are supported by sufficient evidence and whether they have a consistent logic. It is important to be rigorous about this, because we tend to view findings that we agree with as more credible.
- Generalisability of the findings: to what extent can the findings be generalised to other settings? For quantitative studies, statistical generalisation is important and this is linked to sampling procedures. For qualitative research, generalisation is not viewed in the same way and the important issue is whether the concepts that are generated are meaningful in other settings. Is the study clear about the extent to which its findings can be generalised to other settings? If so, does this seem reasonable given the limitations of the study?

- Research ethics: how does the study address ethical issues? This should include ethical procedures followed and address issues such as informed consent, ethical data management and how potential risks were avoided. It can also include discussion of the values that underpin the study.

Not all of the literature you identify will be research studies. They may be opinion pieces in which the authors put forward a particular argument or viewpoint based upon their experience or on previous literature. However, many of the same criteria are relevant. Is the argument plausible? What evidence do the authors provide to substantiate their claims? Sometimes you may find an article that provides a literature review of your topic area. This may be useful for understanding the key issues and authors. However, do not assume that the authors are coming from an impartial perspective. They may have an allegiance to a particular point of view or position and, consequently, they may place less emphasis on, or even ignore, literature that does not support their stance.

A number of frameworks for critiquing literature of all kinds, including empirical research studies, clinical guidelines and systematic reviews and meta-analyses, are available. Some useful websites are suggested at the end of this chapter.

Documentary analysis

This section discusses documentary analysis, which is one of the lesser known and used social research methods; it appears similar to a literature search but is quite different.

Documentary analysis is likely to become more popular in the future because the increasing availability of online documents means that significantly more data are readily available. Indeed, digital archives could revolutionise some research forms such as historical studies in a way equalled only by the invention of printing (McCulloch, 2004, page 41).

This section introduces you to a process of undertaking a documentary analysis, using the example of a case study to illustrate the process. Issues in choosing documentary analysis as a method for proposals will be discussed in this chapter, and issues in analysis will be discussed in Chapter 5.

First of all, what do we mean by a 'document'? The question of what constitutes a document is interpreted in an increasingly wide variety of ways; for example, not just paper documents, but visual data such as photographs and television programmes. Consequently, the term 'text' rather than document has been used to include a wider variety of material (O'Leary, 2004).

The significant growth in online material has provided rich new sources of data. Subject-based discussion groups or bulletin boards provide interesting material but raise new ethical dilemmas. For example, service users and carers use bulletin boards anonymously as a way of accessing support and sharing experiences. Although the information is public and usually anonymous, the individuals cannot be considered to have consented to have their information used for research purposes. These ethical dilemmas are likely to become more acute as more online material becomes available.

Documents are central to the everyday realities of working in the healthcare field and serve many purposes. Legislative and policy statements issued by governmental departments set out the principles and priorities of the current administration and their development is recorded through the parliamentary process. Inquiry reports investigate individual cases where things have gone seriously wrong and make recommendations for the future. Media documents in print, online and audiovisual forms record events that can shape public opinions about health and social care issues. Governance documents, such as committee minutes, record key discussions and decisions made about resource allocation and other key decisions. Individual case records document events and processes and record decision making by different professionals, including nurses. All of these are legitimate sources for documentary analysis.

Documents not only passively record events, but can have a profound influence on the ways that we understand and structure those events. When you go out to conduct a patient assessment, it is likely that the documentation that you complete will influence how you see the service user, your role and the function of your service. This too is a legitimate focus for research and can identify implicit beliefs and assumptions contained within documents.

Scott (1990) outlines four criteria for judging documents for research purposes. The first criterion is authenticity, which focuses on issues of soundness and authorship. We need to establish the authenticity of the document and the identity of the author. For example, government documents and inquiry reports may be published under the name of a minister or chairperson but may be the work of a team of people (Scott, 1990).

The second criterion is credibility, which focuses on sincerity and accuracy. We must consider the extent to which a document is likely to be an undistorted account. No account will be entirely undistorted, because decisions have been made about what to include or what to leave out as well as how the material will be presented. The task is to establish the extent to which the author had a clear interest in presenting material in a certain light. For example, both government policy documents and nursing reports share the dual functions of informing readers and also persuading them about the wisdom of the course of action proposed.

The third criterion is representativeness, which focuses on the extent to which the documents available are representative of all documents (whether the document is typical of its kind). For historical documents, this can include asking whether some documents survived while others did not. It can also raise issues of power; for example, when a service user goes to see a psychiatrist, it will usually be the psychiatrist who documents the encounter. Similarly, meetings can involve considerable debate, but the version that is presented in the minutes would usually have precedence.

The final criterion is meaning, which focuses on whether the evidence is clear and comprehensible. It is also important to establish whether the meanings contained within a document are literal or whether they are latent (Scott, 1990). Literal meanings are explicit and straightforward, whilst latent meanings are implicit and require further interpretation.

The research question and approach will influence how you approach your documents. If it is a traditional, positivist approach, documents may be seen as providing straightforward evidence for social phenomena. For example, newspaper articles may provide evidence of the frequency and severity of attacks by people diagnosed with schizophrenia on members of the public. If your research approach is interpretative, documents may be interpreted as reflecting how social phenomena have been constructed. The same newspaper articles would be viewed, but the interpretation and analysis are different.

Common pitfalls

The relatively infrequent use of documentary analysis is at least partly due to the confusion about how to complete a documentary analysis. One of the most common problems that students experience is confusing a documentary analysis with a literature review. Sometimes students think that they are doing a documentary analysis because they are reviewing the previous academic and practitioner research on their chosen topic. In fact, they are completing a literature review, which is required in every traditional research proposal and dissertation. This confusion is understandable because students will be analysing documents. However, although superficially similar, documentary analysis is used in a more restricted sense.

A literature review is a critical summary of what other researchers have found (i.e. their analysis of their data). So a literature review reports what other people have found. A documentary analysis is an analysis of data which reports findings from an investigation.

The key to understanding how a documentary analysis differs from a literature review lies in the distinction between primary and secondary sources. A *primary source* is raw data collected to analyse for a research topic whilst a *secondary source* is someone else's analysed data that would form part of your literature review. An analogy would be the study of gender in the paintings of Picasso – the paintings themselves would be primary sources to be analysed, whilst the writings of other commentators would be secondary sources to be discussed in a literature review.

Case study: Documentary analysis

Sarah is a student on a mental health placement. She is aware of how people with mental health problems can experience considerable stigma and discrimination (Green et al., 2002, 2003). She is interested in how the media portrays women with a diagnosis of schizophrenia and has decided to use documentary analysis for her research project within a feminist paradigm.

Sarah has decided to use documentary analysis for several reasons. First, it has lower ethical risks than other methods and usually does not require ethical approval if using publicly available data. Second, it does not require her to gain access to participants. Third, it is easy to collect data, especially if using online sources. This enables more data to be collected and more time for analysis. Finally, the data already exist and are not biased by the researcher in the same way as can happen in interviews and focus groups.

Activity 2.2	*Critical thinking*

Sarah has the documents listed below. Which document is included in the literature review and which document is going to be studied in the documentary analysis?

1. An article from the *Times Online* about a young man with a diagnosis of schizophrenia who was involved in a dispute with a neighbour.
2. A book that describes research into how people with mental health problems are portrayed in the media.

There is a brief outline answer at the end of the chapter.

The distinction between primary and secondary data can occasionally become blurred because it is not only what type of documents are used, but the way in which they are used. For example, a research project about how drug users and their health are portrayed in government policy would be analysing government policy documents as primary sources but also discussing them in a literature review. However, the main secondary sources are likely to be commentators who present their own analyses of how drug users and their health are viewed within society.

The process of conducting a documentary analysis has three stages:

1. deciding on a research question and designing a plan;
2. deciding which documents to analyse and what to include in the sample;
3. collecting and analysing your data.

The first two stages will be discussed in this chapter, and stage three in Chapter 5.

Stage 1: Research question and study design

Most research methods are located within a particular tradition; for example, surveys and questionnaires within the quantitative tradition, interviews within the qualitative tradition. Documentary analysis is unusually versatile in that both quantitative and qualitative research designs can be used.

Research summary

One of the research studies that Sarah found for her literature review was a study about how people with mental health problems are represented in the media.

The Glasgow Media Group produced a classic study into media portrayals of people with mental health problems (Philo, 1996). In order to identify the dominant messages which are being given out about mental illness across a variety of media, the study included all media content for a period of one month. The sample included television news and press reporting, popular magazines, children's literature, soap operas, films and dramas.

(Continued)

(Continued)

The study yielded a total of 562 items whose content fell into five main categories:

1. violence to others;
2. harm to self;
3. prescriptive/advice;
4. criticism of accepted definitions of mental illness;
5. 'comic' images.

The authors found that the category of 'violence to others' was by far the most common, outweighing the next most common ('advice') by a ratio of almost four to one. They also found that items linking mental illness and violence tended to receive 'headline' treatment, while more sympathetic items were largely 'back page' in their profile, such as problem page letters or health columns. For an excellent update on media representations of mental health, see Clements and Foster (2008).

Having read the Glasgow study, Sarah has decided that *content analysis* would be a suitable method for her research. Content analysis is a way of analysing documents and texts by measuring the frequency and prominence of specific words or phrases.

Advantages and disadvantages of documentary analysis

Documentary analysis has a number of advantages and disadvantages as a research method. One of the main advantages is that the data already exist so it is a matter of gaining access rather than collecting data. It is an attractive research method because it avoids the time-consuming process of negotiating access to participants and arranging interviews or focus groups. This makes it economical to collect data, in both cost and time. This is particularly true if using documents in electronic form because text organisation is easier and search engines enable quick location of items of interest. Since the documents already exist independently, they cannot be biased by the researcher in the same way as interviews and focus groups.

As with all research designs, consideration needs to be given to ethical concerns and documentary analysis should not be considered an ethically neutral process (McCulloch, 2004). However, it presents lower ethical risks than other methods because it does not directly involve participants. Consequently, ethical approval is often not required if you are using publicly available data. The highest risks relate to the use of sensitive information, such as client information, but issues around copyright, freedom of information and data protection need to be addressed by all research projects.

The availability of data means that it is easy to become overwhelmed by the amount of information and to find it difficult to decide what to leave out. Since an analysis of data occurs outside the original context in which the document was produced, the framework that was used to create the original document may be significantly different from the framework that would be used to analyse it. Whilst this may produce valuable insights, it can be challenging.

Documents available may be limited both in scope and in quality, or may not focus solely on the issue you are interested in. The quality of the documents may be variable and, if they are in different formats, they may be difficult to compare and may require considerable preparation before they can be analysed. For example, if you were comparing a child death inquiry report from the 1970s with a modern inquiry report, the quality, detail and format of the documents are likely to be quite different (Parton, 2004). There may be omissions and inaccuracies in the original documents and some documents may be more likely to survive than others. Although bias cannot be introduced into what is contained within the documents, personal biases may influence which types of records are used and their interpretation. These issues do not preclude using documentary analysis, but would require discussing in your proposal or dissertation.

Stage 2: Deciding which documents to analyse and what to include in a sample

Applying sampling concepts to documentary analysis requires the development of clear rules about what should be included in the sample, known as inclusion criteria. These criteria identify what is a suitable document and exclude documents that fall outside a study, and should be acknowledged in proposals and dissertations.

Activity 2.3	*Critical thinking*

In the case study, Sarah is interested in how newspapers have portrayed women with a diagnosis of schizophrenia. What inclusion criteria should Sarah use for her study?

There is a brief outline answer at the end of the chapter.

One of the most common questions is 'what is an acceptable sample size?' Documentary analysis is one of the research methods that has the greatest variability in sample size because the documents themselves are so variable. Government policy documents or inquiry reports can be several hundred pages long and the sample size will be different compared to analysing short newspaper articles. Consequently, this issue needs to be discussed with supervisors and outlined in proposals.

What if there are too many or too few documents?

A common difficulty is having too many or too few documents to choose from. To some extent, this can be controlled through inclusion criteria, either by narrowing the criteria to reduce the number of documents or by widening the criteria to increase the number of documents included in the sample. In the case study, Sarah could reduce or increase the number of documents by looking for a shorter or longer time period or she could change other criteria, such as including feature articles as well as news items.

However, this approach can distort the sample. For example, Sarah could pick a short time period and this could coincide with a major news story about a person diagnosed with schizophrenia, which would present a significantly different picture to another time period. A commonly used alternative approach when you have too many documents is to use random sampling, which is particularly appropriate for content analysis. Random sampling involves making a selection of cases (the sample) from the whole group of possible cases (the population) on the basis of chance. In random sampling, each case has an equal chance of being selected.

In Sarah's case, she completed an electronic search and found that there were 600 news articles involving people diagnosed with schizophrenia during 2013. Since this is too large a number to analyse, she decided to select a 10% sample randomly, namely 60 articles. She could do this through a random number table or through an online random number generator (such as www.randomizer.org). Having obtained 60 random numbers between 1 and 600, she would select the articles from her search that corresponded with these numbers.

If there are too few documents, a more qualitative analysis may be appropriate, depending on the research question. In Chapter 5, qualitative approaches to data analysis such as thematic analysis will be outlined and these may be more appropriate. Documents in electronic format are much easier to analyse.

Case study: Preliminary searches

Sarah decided to use ProQuest, a national electronic database of newspaper articles from a range of national tabloid and broadsheet newspapers. The ProQuest database includes the Daily Mail, Daily Telegraph, Guardian, Times *and* Independent *newspapers. This was available through her university library and enabled her to undertake a preliminary search to establish how much material is available.*

In order to undertake her preliminary search, she must decide which search terms to use. Since she is searching for articles that refer to individuals diagnosed with schizophrenia, she used the search term 'schizo*'. The Boolean operator '*' is a wildcard, which means that all phrases that include the word stem 'schizo' (e.g. schizophrenia, schizophrenic), will be included. She considered using wider terms such as 'mental health', but a preliminary search retrieved a very large number of articles that rarely related specifically to schizophrenia.

She found that there are approximately 50 articles per month that refer to individuals diagnosed with schizophrenia, spread evenly over the year. Looking at a one-year time period, the search returned 600 articles spread evenly throughout the year. Sarah randomly chose a 10% sample (60 articles) over the year. If it were a topic that was likely to show variations throughout the year, e.g., news coverage of sunburn, then an alternative would be systematic sampling focusing upon specific time periods.

> *The articles that Sarah identified took two days to code, working on the basis of approximately 10–15 minutes per article. Once Sarah had identified a suitable article, she was able to store it ready for analysis, making sure that she kept details of the source and date of the article.*

Chapter summary

This chapter began by defining what is meant by a literature review and exploring its roles and functions. The process of undertaking a literature search was reviewed, focusing on the challenge of finding high-quality material in your topic area.

The procedures for undertaking a literature search and making effective notes were examined. You were asked to consider what it means to analyse critically the literature that you find and clear guidelines have been discussed.

We then examined how to undertake a documentary analysis, making the point that, although superficially similar, there are key differences between a documentary analysis and a literature review.

Activity answers

Activity 2.1: Critical thinking (literature searches) (page 33)

Joan is already clear about her research question, namely, 'What is best practice in caring for diabetic leg ulcers?' For her, the key words 'diabetic feet' and 'diabetic leg ulcer care' were relevant; she realised that 'diabetes' alone would be unmanageably large. She added 'treatment' and 'research' to limit the search to these areas only. She wanted to include literature from outside the UK but was aware that she would need to restrict it to material in English, as this was her only language. Her PICO was as follows:

- population: diabetics;
- intervention: leg ulcer care;
- control (comparison): dressing types;
- outcome: healing rates.

Activity 2.2: Critical thinking (documentary analysis) (page 41)

1. The article is a primary source – raw data about how the media portrays people with mental health problems.
2. The book is a secondary source – a developed analysis based upon the author's own research, which Sarah needs to discuss in her literature review.

Activity 2.3: Critical thinking (inclusion criteria) (page 43)

In the case study, the inclusion criteria would be that the articles are news articles, rather than other forms of articles, such as features. The articles must relate to an individual diagnosed with schizophrenia, which must be used in a clinical sense, not a colloquial or metaphorical sense (e.g. not 'his performance on the football pitch was schizophrenic'). Sarah has decided that she will use only articles from the latest full year.

Further reading

Literature reviews

Aveyard, H (2014) *Doing a Literature Review in Health and Social Care: A Practical Guide*, 3rd edition. Berkshire: Open University Press.
A useful and rigorous account of conducting a literature review.

Cullum, N, Ciliska, D, Haynes, B and Marks, S (2007) *Evidence-Based Nursing: An Introduction*. Oxford: WileyBlackwells.
A useful and interesting guide to understanding evidence-based practice in nursing.

Ellis, P (2013) *Evidence-Based Practice in Nursing*, 2nd edition. London: Sage/Learning Matters.
More detailed information about evidence-based practice in nursing.

Fink, A (2005) *Conducting Research Literature Reviews: From the Internet to Paper*, 2nd edition. London: Sage.
A useful guide which focuses on evaluating quantitative research and provides an outline of appropriate statistical tests when appraising research evidence.

Greenhalgh, T (2010) *How to Read a Paper*, 3rd edition. London: BMJ Publishing.
A book-length guide to appraising research papers from both quantitative and qualitative traditions.

Greenhalgh, T and Taylor, R (1997) How to read a paper: papers that go beyond numbers (qualitative research). *British Medical Journal*, 315: 740–743.
A classic article that provides a clear account of evaluating qualitative research studies.

Hart, C (1998) *Doing a Literature Review: Releasing the Social Science Research Imagination*. London: Sage.
A classic introduction to compiling your literature review that gives detailed guidance on structure and evaluating arguments.

Documentary analysis

Atkinson, P and Coffey, A (2004) Analysing documentary realities, in Silverman, D (ed.) *Qualitative Research: Theory, Method and Practice*, 2nd edition. London: Sage.
Interesting and useful discussion about documentary analysis from a qualitative perspective.

Epstein, I (2010) *Clinical Data-Mining: Integrating Practice and Research*. Oxford: Oxford University Press.
An excellent and interesting account of a new approach to documentary analysis, including practical examples of previous clinical data-mining studies. An insightful and entertaining read, likely to become a classic.

Prior, L (2003) *Using Documents in Social Research*. London: Sage.
Detailed account of documentary analysis from a qualitative perspective. Interesting discussion of the philosophical basis for documentary analysis.

Scott, J (1990) *A Matter of Record: Documentary Sources in Social Research*. Cambridge: Polity Press.
A classic text in documentary analysis, concentrating mainly on historical documents.

Useful websites

http://ethos.bl.uk/Home.do
British Library search engine for searching for PhD theses.

www.casp-uk.net
The Critical Appraisal Skills Programme (CASP) has developed the following tools to help with the process of critically appraising articles:

- systematic reviews;
- randomised controlled trials (RCTs);
- qualitative research;
- economic evaluation studies;
- cohort studies;
- case-control studies;
- diagnostic test studies;
- clinical prediction rules.

www.evidence.nhs.uk/default.aspx
NHS Evidence provides a database of publications for health and social care practitioners.

www.jrf.org.uk
The Joseph Rowntree Foundation is a national research and development charity that funds a range of research into social policy.

www.socialresearchmethods.net
The Web Center for Social Research Methods is a USA-based resource that provides useful material, including content on choosing appropriate statistical tests and concept mapping.

www.vts.intute.ac.uk
Intute Virtual Training Suite is based at Bristol University and provides online training to enable you to make the most effective use of online resources for nursing courses.

Chapter 3
Planning your research proposal or dissertation

Chapter aims

After reading this chapter, you should be able to:

- plan the stages of your research project;
- choose your research area or topic, and develop your research question with the help of concept maps;
- draw up a timetable for carrying out your research, and a list of resource issues;
- understand the basic ethical principles governing research, and how to seek approval for your study.

Introduction

This chapter looks at how you go about planning your research proposal or dissertation. We take you through the key issues: planning the stages of the research process; choosing your research area/topic and developing your research question using concept maps; developing a research plan and timetable and considering resource issues; and addressing ethical approval and research governance issues.

Planning your research

Planning your research properly takes time but this is an essential step which will help you to construct a convincing argument about why the research is worth doing and how you will do it. It is important in your planning to allow yourself sufficient time to undertake your research and allow for possible delays. For example, common delays occur when trying to obtain ethical approvals, or if participants cancel and you have to rearrange appointments. Similarly, transcribing interviews or focus groups takes longer than people anticipate and data analysis even more so, so this all needs to be reflected in the planning and timetabling of activities. As a novice researcher it would be worthwhile keeping a research journal or logbook in which you could jot down ideas, notes of material you have read, conversations that you have had and to-do lists. Postgraduate students are likely to be asked to keep a portfolio-type research log which will contain all this information and be used at supervision meetings with supervisors. You could record all of your thoughts as your proposal develops and include the texts that you identify and the results of your literature searches. It would be invaluable in promoting reflexivity, as it enables you to capture and examine your thoughts on the research process, the decisions that you have made and your role as researcher. This is a particularly important process in qualitative research, and should be built into qualitative proposals. There are six stages in research (see Table 3.1) which we will now explore in detail.

Phase	Stage
Phase 1: Planning	Stage 1: Choosing your research topic and formulating your research question
	Stage 2: Choosing your research approach. This will be the main focus of this chapter and consists of the following stages:
	• deciding your research approach, qualitative and quantitative research • deciding your research design, including research method and sampling
	Stage 3: Undertaking the literature review
Phase 2: Data	Stage 4: Collecting your data
Phase 3: Data analysis and writing it up	Stage 5: Analysing your data. Making sense of the data that you obtain will be discussed in Chapter 7
	Stage 6: Writing up your research

Table 3.1: The six stages of research

Choosing your research topic and formulating your research question

The initial stage of the research process is choosing a research topic and developing it into a specific research question. Do not be tempted to formulate complicated questions on the basis that they sound academic. If you read classic research studies, you will find that they have worked well because they have chosen simple, focused research questions.

Your first task is to identify a research topic and formulate your research questions. While the former is often quite easy, the latter can be quite challenging. This is because most students have one or more general areas of interest but translating this into specific research questions usually involves reformulation.

When choosing your research topic, there are three main considerations:

1. *What are you interested in studying?* You may choose a subject to research for a range of reasons, such as personal or professional experience, an interest in the academic subject and an awareness of a gap in the literature. Choose a subject that you are genuinely interested in, otherwise it is difficult to maintain enthusiasm over an extended period. Remember that this is likely to be the part of your course where you have the greatest freedom to choose what you study. Even though you may not undertake the research,

remember that you will need to spend a lot of time searching literature and critiquing it, and drafting and redrafting a final form of words, so you need to be able to maintain your enthusiasm. At this point, you should also be clear about the aims and be able to justify why the topic is worth pursuing.

2. *What will fit your course requirements?* You need to familiarise yourself with the expectations of your institution about the format and scope of your research proposal. Do not underestimate the importance of this, since your overall aim is to complete your nursing degree and this will only happen if your research proposal meets the course requirements, however good it may be.

3. *What are you able to study?* There are several components to addressing what it is possible to study. First, what can you research ethically? You need to consider how your research might impact on your participants and other stakeholders, if you were actually to undertake it, even if you are only writing a proposal. This will need to be discussed in detail in the proposal, concentrating on ethical principles rather than simply saying 'ethical approval will be gained prior to commencing the research'. Second, what do you have the time and resources to study? An old adage for a research project is: 'Think about what you want to do. Halve it, then halve it again and you may still struggle to get it all done.' Although you must consider the logistics of the proposal, 'scientific' justifications for sample sizes and recruitment strategies will be more impressive than saying 'this is a small project so I can only interview four people'. Third, what can you get access to study? Many research projects will require you to gain access to participants and you need to consider how practical this is; this should be acknowledged in the proposal.

It is important that your research question is not so broad that it is unrealistic for you to be able to answer it, nor so narrow that it lacks sufficient substance. It is more common for students to have difficulties because their research questions are too broad, rather than too narrow. Students often write proposals with lots of aims and objectives, which in reality would be too complex to undertake: discuss it fully with your supervisor but stick with one or two aims and two or three objectives at the most. A common pitfall that nursing students make is to state as an aim or objective that they want to change practice. This is laudable but unless the project is specifically designed to change practice, such as in an action research design, it is unlikely to change anything and the best you can hope for is to inform practice or make recommendations.

A traditional recommendation from research supervisors is to be wary of choosing research topics that have attracted recent media attention. The rationale for this is that you are likely to find a considerable amount of media coverage, but little research or academic writing. The danger is that the final dissertation or proposal will reproduce the generalisations and stereotyping presented in the media reports with little evidence from research studies or academic writing. However, some topics do have a reasonable academic literature and the student may be interested in investigating how the topic has been portrayed in the media. In this case, media coverage would be a legitimate source of data for a documentary analysis (see Chapter 2).

Why formulate an overall research question?

A clear question forms your aims and objectives, drives your choice of methodology and methods, and if you were actually to undertake the research it would require you to write up how the question was answered in the discussion section.

So, it is important to formulate an overall research question because it will focus your choice of research design and your literature search. It is all too easy to find yourself going in several different directions during a literature search or to collect too much unfocused data and then become confused about what to include and what to leave out.

You may find that you have more than one overall research question. If so, they need to link well to form an overall research project. If you find that you have two entirely separate research questions, you probably have two research projects and you need to decide which one you want to undertake.

Choosing your research approach and design: quantitative and qualitative research

Once you have formulated an initial research topic, you need to consider which research approach and research methods to propose. As we discussed in Chapter 1, social research has traditionally been divided into quantitative and qualitative approaches. These approaches have different views about the nature of knowledge and different methods and priorities. Although this distinction is contested (Layder, 1993), it is commonly used and there is little evidence of it abating completely (Bryman, 2012).

Some examples of student projects using quantitative approaches

Here are some examples of student research proposals using a quantitative approach.

Case study: Questionnaires

Varsha is a final-year student who is interested in her fellow students' experiences of their nursing education. She proposes to use questionnaires to study her fellow students' attitudes towards their professional training, particularly whether they feel it is preparing them for the realities of working as qualified nurses. She is interested in whether participants' responses differ according to year of study, age, gender and amount of pre-qualifying experience. For example, Varsha has a hypothesis that older students will report higher levels of confidence in their ability to practise and wants to test this out. See Chapter 6 on questionnaires for a full discussion of this example.

Case study: Documentary analysis

Sarah is a student on a mental health placement. She is interested in how the media portrays women with a diagnosis of schizophrenia and has decided to use documentary analysis for her research project within a feminist paradigm. She could use either a quantitative or qualitative approach, but chooses to use a quantitative method called content analysis. This is a data analysis method that uses objective and systematic counting and recording procedures to produce quantitative data about the manifest (i.e. visible) content of communication. Sarah decided to use an electronic database of newspaper articles from a range of national tabloid and broadsheet newspapers to study coverage of mental health over a one-year period.

Some examples of student projects using qualitative approaches

Case study: Focus group

Patrick is a child health nursing student on placement in a large, local authority family centre. He is interested in social workers' views on the barriers to fathers being involved in parenting assessments.

Patrick decided that a focus group would be a good research method because it would enable him to hear a range of views, and participants to interact with each other and challenge one another's views. Patrick's focus is on participants' professional experience rather than their personal biographies and it would take much longer to conduct interviews that would produce a similar amount of data. The disadvantages of focus groups are that it can be difficult to arrange for a group of people to meet, and the possibility that some group members will not feel able to express their opinions.

Patrick considered how to select his participants and how many focus groups to run. Eight staff members were interested in being involved and Patrick contacted a neighbouring family centre and managed to recruit eight staff members, which would enable him to run two focus groups.

Case study: Interviews

Victoria is a mental health student on placement in a voluntary sector mental health organisation. She is interested in how voluntary sector staff view work in partnership with statutory sector mental health organisations and would like to use qualitative interviews to explore this further.

Victoria must decide who to include in her sample. She considers that the most appropriate strategy would be purposive sampling, in which she selects participants who are most likely to yield useful information. This is often based upon factors such as the participant's knowledge, experience or role. She decides to interview two groups of voluntary sector staff, one working in her placement agency and another in a similar voluntary organisation in a neighbouring area. She will focus on staff members who are likely to experience partnership working as part of their everyday role.

Do I really have to discuss epistemology?

In the last two chapters, we have discussed some of the main epistemological positions that have influenced quantitative and qualitative approaches. A common student question is whether it is necessary to talk about epistemology in your final dissertation or proposal. The extent to which you are expected to be explicit about your epistemological position depends upon whether you are completing an undergraduate or postgraduate degree and the requirements of your individual institution. Most postgraduate taught courses like Master's degrees require you to discuss in significant detail your epistemological position, while doctoral students would expect this to be a major element of their work. Undergraduate courses may not, but this varies between institutions. In undergraduate nursing programmes it is likely that some discussion of the underlying philosophical issues surrounding a qualitative or quantitative approach will be an impressive feature of your work and is likely to score higher marks than if it is largely ignored.

Either way, the important point is to not be intimidated by the terminology, but to read around the different approaches and make sure the approach you choose is reasoned as it determines your data collection methods: the research question dictates the epistemological position, which indicates the methods of data collection and analysis, rather than the other way around. Students may think they want to 'do qualitative research because it's easier', but this may not be possible for some questions, like comparisons between treatments.

Imagine that your epistemological position, design and research methods are like different items of clothing. For example, if you choose a qualitative approach with an interpretative epistemology, then choose a highly structured questionnaire; this is similar to choosing clothes that clash with each other. While each item may be acceptable individually, the combination does not work as they are incompatible, and would lead a tutor to suspect that you did not really understand what you were talking about. Making the different items match is an important part of making your proposal credible.

Moving from a research topic to a specific research question

For some research projects, the transition from having a research topic to formulating a specific research question is smooth and unproblematic. For others, it can take considerable time to narrow down the research topic and this is usually something that happens in parallel with developing the literature review. When you see how others have approached your research topic and the range of methodologies they have used, this is likely to focus your thinking.

A useful tool or technique to aid this process is the concept map, which is a way of visually representing the different elements of your topic. Concept mapping allows you to think about your research topic because it helps you to break down your topic into its constituent parts and examine them in more depth.

Case study: Concept mapping

As Patrick's interest is in safeguarding children, he wants to propose an investigation into how childcare social workers engage fathers when there are child welfare concerns. However, he is unclear how he is going to narrow this topic down to a research question.

Patrick decides to use a concept map to identify the different angles from which he could approach this topic.

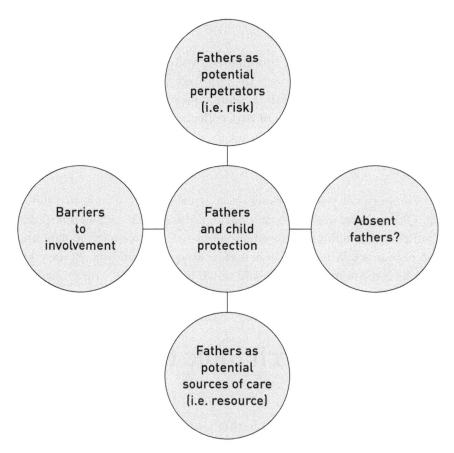

Figure 3.1: Initial concept map

Having completed his initial concept map (Figure 3.1), Patrick decided that he was interested in identifying possible barriers to fathers' involvement.

Activity 3.1   *Critical thinking*

Write your research area at the centre of a piece of paper and map out the possible topics or angles from which you could approach it. Your aim is to move from a general topic area to a specific research question.

Comment

This can be useful to help you check your current understanding of your research topic. When you first do this, your concept map will represent your initial understanding of the topic. As you identify literature, you can update your concept map to create a visual representation of what material is available. You may find that there is a concentration of literature on particular topics, while other topics receive scant discussion. This will influence your choice and can be a useful subject for discussion in your literature review.

As this is your personal map, there is no outline at the end of the chapter.

Timetabling and resources

A coherent proposal gives a plan of what you intend to investigate and how you intend to go about it. It needs a timetable to show that you have considered all the steps necessary and allocated sufficient time to each. The key stages in a research proposal are as follows:

- ethics application and approval;
- literature review;
- recruitment;
- data collection;
- data analysis;
- writing up;
- dissemination.

Each of these needs to be allocated time. You may also want to include project meetings and time for writing your journal or reflective log. Proposals are generally planned with activities scheduled monthly rather than weekly. The timeframe depends on your deadlines or coursework requirements; in reality this would depend on project funding, but for an undergraduate proposal this would not be a consideration. Designing a timetable can be done simply using a table in Microsoft Word (Figure 3.2): use the Table function under the Insert tab, then shade the relevant months when the activities will be undertaken. This is a highly simplified example of how a proposal might be planned, and in reality the stages would be more overlapping, with activities not necessarily carried out in such a delineated fashion. More complex and more interesting designs can be made using Gantt charts.

Activity	Sept	Oct	Nov	Dec	Jan	Feb	March	April	May
Ethics application and approval	▓	▓							
Literature review	▓	▓	▓						
Recruitment			▓						
Data collection				▓	▓				
Data analysis					▓	▓	▓		
Writing up								▓	▓
Dissemination									▓
Project meetings	▓	▓	▓	▓	▓	▓	▓	▓	▓
Reflective journaling	▓	▓	▓	▓	▓	▓	▓	▓	▓

Figure 3.2: Simple project planning using a Microsoft Word table

Resources

What will you need to help you to conduct the research? As a student writing a proposal, you are in the fortunate position of not having to think too much about the practicalities of this issue, but you may be asked to give an indication of the sorts of things you think you would need. In reality, the majority of research projects are entirely dependent on external funding from charities or government research organisations: they will not occur without it. Universities employ staff to conduct research as a result of getting external funding – they rarely fund studies from internal sources, and professors spend hours writing proposals and chasing funding bids. This is a highly competitive process and careers are made as a result of obtaining large amounts of money. Nowadays, a system known as full economic costing (FEC) governs the estimates of sums of money included in bids that universities make. The University of Oxford site shows how they operationalise FEC (www.admin.ox.ac.uk/fec). Costing bids to external sources is a complex business and universities employ finance staff specifically for this purpose. Don't think about doing it yourself, as it's very difficult to get it right!

Activity 3.2   *Critical thinking*

In order to plan your resources, think through the sorts of things you think you would need for your project. Is this staff, computers, training, office space? Write down on a piece of paper what resources you will need.

There is a brief outline answer at the end of the chapter.

Dissemination

For a proposal you would not need to use any strategies for dissemination, but might be asked to write about what you would do. There is an argument that conducting research purely for one's own purposes is unethical, and while undergraduate students are unlikely to have pressure put on them to publish their findings if they do undertake empirical research, postgraduate students will certainly be expected to do so. This is because findings contribute to a body of knowledge, even if it is a small contribution, and this body of knowledge may eventually become sufficient for changes in practice to be recommended. In general, dissemination would include publishing findings in journals. There is a distinction between good academic journals such as the *Journal of Advanced Nursing* and the *International Journal of Nursing Studies*, which have international reputations and readerships as publishers of research findings, and professional journals such as the *Nursing Times*, which aim to inform practice. It is quite hard to be published in academic journals, and you would need help from an experienced author to achieve this, but professional journals are usually slightly easier. As well as publishing in journals, you would need to write a project report. You could also present your findings at conferences. Although this may be scary at first, you get a great sense of achievement from it, and probably a couple of nights in a nice venue while you attend the conference!

Addressing ethical issues and research governance

An important part of planning your research project is addressing ethical issues and following ethical governance processes. Each university has its own system of ethics committees and there are also similar processes within the NHS and other statutory agencies such as local authorities to protect patients, service users and staff from unethical research practices. As registrants, or potential registrants, with a professional body like the Nursing and Midwifery Council (NMC), we also have a duty to abide by its code of conduct, and this overrides the fact that a student may be acting as a researcher: a nurse's first duty is to protect patients and clients at all times, and this should be acknowledged in proposals. If NMC registrants uncover issues of serious professional misconduct this must be passed on to the relevant authorities.

The NHS research ethics procedure is the most well known, and as a general rule any research proposal which intends to use NHS staff, patients/clients or facilities must be submitted for approval using the NHS system. This is called the NHS Research Ethics Service (NRES), which is part of the National Patient Safety Agency (NPSA). NRES lists on its website the following mission statement and procedures:

- to protect the rights, safety, dignity and well-being of research participants; and
- to facilitate and promote ethical research that is of potential benefit to participants, science and society.

This is achieved by:

- providing robust and responsive ethical review of research through research ethics committees (RECs);
- providing ethical guidance to RECs;
- providing and delivering a managed structure to support RECs;
- delivering a quality assurance (QA) framework;

- delivering a training programme;
- working with colleagues across the UK to maintain a UK-wide framework for ethical review;
- working with colleagues in the wider regulatory environment to streamline the processes for approving research;
- promoting and supporting transparency in research.

Since 2011, there have been changes to the types of study that need to go before a full NHS REC. REC review is required if a research project involves humans (NHS patients, their relatives or carers, healthy volunteers) and/or the collection of human tissue. Research involving any of the following requires NHS REC review:

- investigational medicinal products;
- non CE-marked medical devices or CE-marked medical devices that have been modified or are being used for a new purpose;
- exposure to ionising radiation;
- people who lack (or lose) the capacity to give informed consent;
- processing of confidential patient information without consent;
- material, consisting of or containing human cells, which has been taken from the living or the deceased;
- midwives conducting a clinical trial;
- prisoners (REC policy, rather than a legal requirement);
- xenotransplantation (REC policy, rather than a legal requirement).

Research involving any of the following no longer requires NHS REC review:

- NHS staff recruited by virtue of their professional role;
- previously collected, non-identifiable tissue samples or information;
- acellular material, e.g. plasma or serum;
- healthcare market research;
- research involving premises and facilities (e.g. research undertaken by a university department on NHS premises, involving healthy volunteers not recruited as NHS patients and not subject to any legal requirements would not require review by an REC).

Applications for ethical approval in the NHS must go through its web-based Integrated Research Application System (IRAS), which is a unified system for applying for permission and approval for NHS research in the UK. In practice, IRAS has developed guidance for interpreting whether a study needs to come before its full committee structure, and it draws a distinction between research, service evaluation and audit (NPSA, 2010). Its definition of research has come to emphasise more experimental designs such as randomised controlled trials which are evaluating new treatments or interventions with patients and clients, and there is also particular scrutiny of research where tissue samples are involved. As such, there is something of a dichotomy in this medical-model understanding of the term 'research' and its need to safeguard vulnerable patients and clients, compared to the understanding of research from a social science perspective, where 'research' means any type of inquiry where the intention is to study something by collecting data and creating new knowledge and/or understanding of that topic. This can work in the favour of nursing researchers because it can mean that their proposals may not actually need full ethical approval through IRAS: projects evaluating the establishment of new services or roles within the NHS may be acceptable for academic awards and be considered 'research' in university departments but may be considered 'service evaluation' by IRAS. Students who are actually required to collect data should discuss this with their supervisors and use the Health Research Authority (HRA) Decision Tool (see useful websites section on page 62). It may be acceptable for students to ask for an opinion from the local NHS committee chair. This would save time and effort as the student would then not need to complete the online IRAS form or go before a full committee. The e-mail address of the committee chair's secretary can be obtained through the local NHS Trust Research and Development Department.

Case study: Ethical approval and service evaluation

Williamson et al. (2010a) conducted a programme of evaluation of their university faculty's Placement Development Teams (PDTs). These PDTs were established to provide better support for students and their mentors in clinical practice settings. They interviewed students and key NHS stakeholders.

This project was deemed as service evaluation by the local NHS committee chair and did not require full ethical approval through IRAS. The chair put this in writing and this was used as evidence when the proposal was submitted to the university faculty ethics committee for approval. The project did, however, require research governance approval from each site in which the research was to be carried out.

All proposals will require some work for them to be acceptable to any committee, including the NHS one, and in your plan you need to allocate at least two months to get ethical approval based on submission deadlines, re-doing and resubmitting the proposal before final approval. Two months is a bare minimum; three is more realistic. You cannot begin recruitment or data collection in any form until full ethical approval is obtained. There is now a process called Proportionate Ethical Review, where researchers are asked to identify if there are 'no material ethical issues' at submission. If there are none, the approval process for these studies is delegated to special subcommittees, which should be quicker and simpler. Information on Proportionate Reviews can be found on the HRA website (www.hra.nhs.uk).

Research governance

Regardless of whether your proposal would need to go to IRAS, you will need to obtain research governance approval from each NHS site in which you plan to collect data, and this must be discussed in your proposal. Research governance approval ensures that your local sites have had scrutiny of, and a chance to comment and make recommendations on, your proposal. Details of how this can be achieved can be obtained through the local Research and Development (R&D) office, which each NHS Trust will have. In addition to this, researchers external to the NHS will need Honorary Contracts with the Trusts in which they plan to conduct research.

University ethics approval

Universities have their own mechanisms for ethical approval, and students should check what these are and acknowledge them in their proposals. If your proposal would need to go to NRES, when approved it will also need to go to your own university faculty ethics committee. Again, this will need to be factored into your timetable. If your proposal does not need to go to NRES, it will still need to be approved by your university.

Non-NHS ethics approval

In 2005 the government introduced the second edition of the Research Governance Framework (Department of Health, 2005) that covers local authorities, and this has made a significant difference in research conducted in local authority areas such as social work. Check out which procedures apply to you at the earliest stages of your research, as you need to consider and discuss them in your project proposal and allow sufficient time to address their requirements in your planning. The Social Care Institute for Excellence (SCIE) also has a research ethics committee, but this does not review student projects.

Ethical principles

The formal consideration of ethical principles came after the Second World War when it came to light that Nazi medical staff had been torturing refugee camp inmates in the name of medical research. Following their convictions at the Nuremberg trials after the war, first the Nuremberg Code (1949) and then the declaration of Helsinki (last revised in 2013 – World Medical Association, 2013) enshrined ethical principles into medical research, and these have been adopted in all research fields.

Activity 3.3   *Evidence-based practice*

List the ethical principles you think are important in research. Use your own language. Then, go to this website on the Nuremberg Code (1949): https://owlspace-ccm. rice.edu/access/content/user/ecy1/Nazi%20Human%20Experimentation/Pages/ the%20code.html. Compare them with those established immediately after the Second World War. Next, go to the Declaration of Helsinki (World Medical Association, 2013) website at www. wma.net/en/30publications/10policies/b3 and do the same comparison.

Comment
The language is different but the basic principles remain unchanged, if updated, between 1949 and 2013.

Although different ethics committees have different practices and priorities, the core principles that ethics committees will be expecting you to address are as follows:

- Non-malevolence: have you taken all reasonable steps to protect your participants from foreseeable harm? For example, interviewing participants can be potentially upsetting and you need to think through how you can ensure they are supported. How will you ensure participants' confidentiality and anonymity?
- Informed consent: you will normally be required to provide written information to potential participants to enable them to make an informed choice.
- Rights to refuse to participate or withdraw without prejudice: if participants do not want to be in the study or change their minds about allowing their data to be used after the event, what arrangements have you made to enable this? Is it clear that if potential participants refuse to take part, they will not be harmed in any way, including receiving less preferential treatment or care from service providers?
- Ethical data management: how will you anonymise your data and who will have access? How will you store the information that you gain? Have you taken reasonable steps to protect your participants from their data being lost?

Chapter summary

This chapter has looked at how you can plan the different stages of research process. It began with some advice on how to choose your research area, narrow it down to a specific topic and then develop your research question. Techniques to help this process, such as using concept maps, were introduced.

The chapter then looked at how you can develop a plan for carrying out your research, including advice on drawing up a timetable. It looked at some of the resource issues that may arise and how you might anticipate them.

Finally, the chapter considered the ethics of research, and the issue of seeking ethical approval from your university or other body.

Activity answer

Activity 3.2: Critical thinking (page 56)

Exactly what you'll need depends on the study. In general you could factor in:

- research assistant(s) – they will do all aspects of the study for you, from recruitment to data collection and analysis;
- computers – essential nowadays;
- office supplies – paper and other equipment;
- website – it is common for there to be a project website nowadays;
- travel expenses for you, your research assistant and participants;
- buy-out – do any of your participants need to be released from work to attend?
- professional or clinical services may be required if there are to be interventions – blood samples may need to be taken and analysed, or there may be more clinic visits;

- refreshments – cups of tea, biscuits and sandwiches may be offered as a thank you or because your interview sessions take place over meal times. Lunch for nurses and students is a reasonable 'perk' and an incentive to attend. Shopping vouchers may also work well.

Further reading

All the books listed below offer good coverage of project-planning issues.

Locke, LF, Spirduso, WW and Silverman, SJ (2007) *Proposals That Work: A Guide for Planning Dissertations and Grant Proposals*, 5th edition. Thousand Oaks, CA: Sage.

Offredy, M and Vickers, P (2010) *Developing a Healthcare Research Proposal: An Interactive Student Guide*. Oxford: WileyBlackwell.

Punch, KF (2006) *Developing Effective Research Proposals*. London: Sage.

Robson, C (2007) *How To Do a Research Project: A Guide for Undergraduate Students*. Oxford: Blackwell Publishing.

Thomas, D and Hodges, ID (2010) *Designing and Planning Your Research Project*. London: Sage.

Walliman, NSR (2005) *Your Undergraduate Dissertation: The Essential Guide for Success*. London: Sage.

Walliman, NSR (2005) *Your Research Project: A Step-by-Step Guide for the First-Time Researcher*. London: Sage.

Useful websites

http://office.microsoft.com/en-us/excel/ha010346051033.aspx
How to create a Gantt chart for a project plan using a Microsoft Excel spreadsheet.

www.crncc.nihr.ac.uk
Website of the National Institute for Health Research Clinical Research Network Coordinating Centre (NIHR CRN CC), which supports clinical research.

www.hra-decisiontools.org.uk/research
Health Research Authority Decision Tool. Guides you about whether your study requires submission to NRES or not.

www.law.umkc.edu/faculty/projects/ftrials/nuremberg/nuremberg.htm
Website on the Nuremberg Trials.

www.nres.nhs.uk
Website of the NHS Research Ethics Service.

www.rdehospital.nhs.uk
An example of the kinds of activities undertaken by a Foundation NHS Trust Research and Development Department. Contains a link to the Research Design Service (www.rds-sw.nihr.ac.uk), which can help with all aspects of project planning and funding applications. Many UK NHS Trusts have similar services which may be accessed locally.

www.wma.net/en/30publications/10policies/b3/index.html
World Medical Association website on the Declaration of Helsinki: Ethical Principles for Medical Research Involving Human Subjects.

Section 3
Using and critiquing research for your final-year project

Chapter 4
Using and critiquing research methods: interviews and focus groups

Chapter aims

After reading this chapter, you should be able to:

- understand how interviews and focus groups can be used as research methods;
- explain how to recruit and select participants for interviews and for focus groups;
- develop an interview schedule and understand the range of interview questions;
- be aware of the difficulties that may arise during focus group sessions.

Introduction

This is the first of five chapters in this section that will introduce you to commonly used research methods and provide an overview of how interviews and focus groups can be understood and how that understanding can contribute to your final-year project or proposal. The emphasis in these chapters is in allowing you to choose the most effective method to use if writing a proposal, rather than in offering a guide to how to use the methods if you were actually undertaking projects for yourself. We will begin by talking about interviews, then move on to looking at focus groups.

Interviews are one of the most popular research methods for nursing researchers and students and feel intuitively 'familiar' because of their use in everyday nursing practice. They are popular in the social sciences generally and are used in the majority of published qualitative research articles (Silverman, 2013). Many research studies use individual interviews to collect data, but focus groups are becoming increasingly popular, and rely on group dynamics to produce data on particular topic areas. They are a form of interview, albeit one with a small group discussing ideas with a facilitator.

In this chapter, you will be asked to consider the advantages and disadvantages of these techniques and when it would be most appropriate to use them. Practical issues raised by their use will be emphasised through case studies and student-centred activities.

Interviews

The interest in interviews is not confined to nursing research. Scourfield (2001) argues that we live in an 'interview culture', in which we are constantly exposed to the idea that something valuable can be learnt by talking one to one with another person. Interviews are intuitively 'human', a face-to-face interaction that enables you to communicate with your participants in depth and offers the opportunity to follow up interesting responses. Interviews can enable people to tell their story and are particularly attractive when researchers want to explore people or communities that have traditionally been ignored, misrepresented or suppressed.

When should interviews be used?

Interviews are best used for research that focuses on the knowledge, values, beliefs and attitudes of participants. They are particularly good at helping participants to think through, consider and make explicit things that have previously been implicit. Robson (2011) argues that facts and behaviour are more easily obtained than beliefs and attitudes, though participants may experience memory lapses or bias so specific questions about things in the present or recent past are best. Questions about a participant's beliefs and attitudes are more complex because responses may be affected by the wording and sequence of questions, but the use of multiple questions and scales can help.

Interviews or questionnaires?

A common dilemma for students is deciding whether to use interviews or questionnaires. The advantages that interviews have over questionnaires is that interviews are good at examining complex issues and producing rich data and they enable participants to discuss sensitive issues in an open way without committing themselves in writing. The disadvantages are that interviews are more time-consuming to complete than questionnaires and it is more complex and time-consuming to analyse interview data.

Interviews or focus groups?

Another dilemma is whether to use interviews or focus groups. While focus groups are effective in accessing shared public knowledge, interviews are fruitful for more personal, biographical information. Interviews can be used in conjunction with focus groups where participants may disclose more sensitive information than they would in a group setting. See the section on focus groups in this chapter for a more detailed discussion.

Types of interview

Although there are a range of different types of interview, the three main forms are structured, unstructured and semistructured interviews.

Structured or standardised interviews

These are highly ordered and tightly designed interviews to collect data that can be quantified. You may have experienced a market research interview, in which multiple-choice questions with a fixed number of responses are used, but such interviews can also be used in the social sciences. Structured interviews have the strength that they are able to produce quantitative data in a clear, readily analysable form. However, they are less popular with students and nursing researchers because the closed nature of questioning does not give them sufficient scope to address more complex, rich, qualitative issues. Structured interviews are part of the quantitative survey research tradition and are similar to questionnaires, which will be discussed in Chapter 6. The remaining forms of interview are generally regarded as part of the qualitative research tradition and form the focus of this chapter.

Unstructured interviews

At the opposite end of the spectrum, unstructured interviews are very open and range from a single question to a list of topics. Sometimes students and nursing researchers consider unstructured interviews because they 'want the data to speak for itself'. Others consider it because they lack confidence in constructing a good *interview schedule* or are unsure about exactly what they want to focus on. The difficulty is that they then produce a number of interview transcripts that are very individual and often do not cover the same ground. This can be a strength for more experienced researchers who are confident in their abilities to analyse diverse and complex data but a real challenge to novice researchers. Consequently, unstructured interviews are best left to the more experienced researcher.

Semistructured interviews

This is the classic structure for qualitative research in the social sciences and the most commonly used format in student research projects. In semistructured interviews, the researcher develops a list of questions, known as an interview schedule. However, there is some flexibility during the interview; for example, if a participant introduces a topic earlier than anticipated, the researcher can change the order of questions. The format is popular because it enables you to have sufficient structure to facilitate data analysis, while giving you sufficient flexibility to explore participants' responses in depth.

Recruiting and selecting participants

One of the most commonly asked questions is *how many people should I plan to interview?* There are usually methodological reasons, such as the achievement of data saturation, which will dictate sampling methods and hence recruitment in qualitative studies using interviews. These issues will need to be explained thoroughly in proposals and adhered to in any actual data collection. While it may also be true that logistical issues such as time constraints and course requirements will influence your recruitment, to list these will not impress supervisors or reviewers with your methodological knowledge and such explanations are best avoided. Consequently, discussing this with your supervisor or tutor is the best first step.

This chapter will focus on sampling strategies for using semistructured or unstructured interviews within a qualitative approach, which is by far the most common approach used in student research projects. If you are planning to employ structured interviews using large sample sizes in a similar way to questionnaires, appropriate sampling strategies will be discussed in depth later.

In qualitative interviewing, the most common approach is non-probability sampling and the specific sampling strategies used are as follows.

Convenience sampling

Convenience sampling (sometimes known as *accidental sampling*) simply means selecting participants based upon the relative ease with which they can be contacted. When planning to use convenience sampling in qualitative research, researchers are not interested in how representative any participant is or whether the participant has particular knowledge or experience. Rather, they are looking for participants who are relatively easy to contact. While this is the least credible of sampling techniques, Bryman (2012) argues that this is far more prevalent than is often recognised in social science research and many quantitative studies and randomised controlled trials in fact use convenience sampling, despite the potential problems associated with it (Williamson, 2003).

Purposive sampling

Purposive sampling (otherwise known as judgemental sampling) is a procedure in which researchers choose participants who, in their judgement, are likely to yield useful information. This is often based upon factors such as the participant's knowledge, experience or role. Interviews are most successful when participants have significant experience in the research topic and are likely to want to discuss it. This is the most commonly used sampling method in student research projects and most writers on qualitative research based on interviews recommend it as the procedure of choice (Bryman, 2012).

Theoretical sampling

Theoretical sampling is an approach, developed as part of grounded theory (Glaser and Strauss, 1967; Strauss and Corbin, 1998), which does not predetermine the number of participants that will be interviewed at the beginning of the study. Instead, researchers will carry on interviewing participants until 'saturation' has been achieved, where no significantly new data are being produced and the themes have been exhausted (Strauss and Corbin, 1998). It has been argued that purposive sampling and theoretical sampling are effectively synonymous (Lincoln and Guba, 1985; Brink, 1991).

Snowball sampling

Snowball sampling is a technique where the researcher selects a small number of participants and asks them to recommend other suitable people who may be willing to participate in the study. This is suitable when participants are difficult to identify and contact, such as sex workers or people who are homeless.

Quota sampling

Quota sampling is a procedure in which the researcher decides to research groups or quotas of people from specific subsections of the total population. Common categories are demographics such as age, gender and ethnicity, but could be related to the research topic. Quota sampling is rarely used in academic research, but it is used frequently in market research (Bryman, 2012).

Case study: Qualitative interviews

Victoria is a nursing student on placement in a voluntary sector mental health organisation. She is interested in how voluntary sector staff view work in partnership with statutory sector mental health organisations and would like to use qualitative interviews to explore this further.

Activity 4.1   *Critical thinking*

Victoria must decide who to include in her sample. Which approach might she choose?

There is a brief outline answer at the end of the chapter.

Ensuring that your data can be analysed

One of your main aims is to ensure that you show that you understand how to analyse data, and that the data will be readily analysable (Arksey and Knight, 1999) if you were to collect them. This cannot be overemphasised, because it is relatively easy to spend time and effort collecting significant amounts of interview data that you later discover are extremely difficult to analyse.

How easy it is to analyse your data depends mainly upon two factors. The first factor depends on how structured your interview will be, since the more structured the interview, the easier it will be to analyse the data you produce (Kvale, 1996). However, a certain amount of flexibility may be appropriate for your research topic. The second factor is how diverse your participants are in terms of experience, role or other issues. One of the most common pitfalls is to choose a sample of participants with such a wide range of roles or backgrounds that the interview data are difficult to analyse. We will discuss qualitative data analysis in more detail in Chapter 5.

Developing an interview schedule

In your project proposal you may be asked to develop a schedule of questions, as this will show how you will go about collecting data which answer your research questions. Your interview schedule is a written plan of how you are going to structure the interview, including what questions you are going to ask and approximately in what order. When developing your interview schedule, your aim is to ensure that your overall research question is answered while promoting a natural flow of conversation that encourages your participants to talk in an open and relaxed way.

Do not be tempted to jot down a few vague ideas and hope that you can muddle through. Without a clear schedule of questions it is likely that, if data were collected, the data would be muddled, take much longer to analyse and not clearly answer the research questions you have decided upon.

During the initial stage of developing an interview schedule, it can be helpful to meet up with a few interested people to generate possible interview questions. Ideally, this would include at least one person who would fit the criteria for your sample because they may spot problems that others may miss. (This could be described as a 'pilot study'.) Likely people to invite could include your practice mentor, placement colleagues and fellow students as well as any party interested in your specific research topic. You should also consider whether service users and carers could be useful in the design stages.

Once you have generated a range of possible questions in the group, take these away to work on them on your own. Review them and discard any that are clearly not relevant. Then divide them into two groups: 'need to know' and 'nice to know' (Krueger and Casey, 2000). 'Need to know' questions are vital to answering your research question, while 'nice to know' questions are ones that you are simply curious about. Be honest and ruthless about this and you will probably be surprised by how many fall into the latter category, leaving you with a schedule of essential questions which you have thought through and are confident about. It may be helpful to arrange another time to meet up with the group when you can test out the questions that you have selected and discuss the order in which they should be asked.

Activity 4.2   *Decision making*

Construct an interview schedule for Victoria (see the case study on page 69). First, construct a question, then think about five relevant questions, then identify which are essential and which are desirable.

There is a brief outline answer at the end of the chapter.

Using vignette questions

An interesting and useful form of questioning is the vignette, which is a simulation of real events depicting hypothetical situations (Wilks, 2004). The most usual way of presenting information is through written material, but alternative formats, such as video material and cartoons, have been used (Wilks, 2004). Vignettes present a scenario to participants, who are then asked about their attitudes, beliefs and responses. For example, in the case study Victoria could present a scenario in which there was a dilemma about interagency working. She could then ask participants how they would react in the scenario and explore the reasoning behind their choices.

The advantage that vignette questions have over more general questions is that they root the question in a specific situation. For example, if general questions are used to ask practitioners how they manage risk when accessing patients or clients, each may respond with broad comments that would be difficult to compare. If the same practitioners are presented with a specific scenario, they are all responding to the same information, so it would be easier to compare their responses. Vignette questions can be particularly effective when dealing with sensitive issues, since vignettes present a hypothetical scenario that can make it less confrontational than asking participants about their own experiences (Finch, 1987).

Vignettes can have more than one stage. For example, a scenario is presented and participants are asked for their immediate responses. They are then presented with further information as the vignette develops and asked about their responses given the new information. This can be used to explore the effects of specific factors.

Advantages and disadvantages of interviews

Interviews have a number of advantages and disadvantages as a research method that you want to employ for your proposal. They may feel intuitively 'familiar' to you because you use them in your everyday nursing practice. You are more likely to have skills and experience of interviews than other research methods and are more likely to feel confident using them. Interviews enable you to access people's feelings and attitudes and allow you to probe for more detailed responses. Consequently, they provide richer and more indepth data. They enable you to follow up interesting responses in ways that are not possible using other methods, such as questionnaires. If you are interested in participants' individual views and experiences, interviews are more likely to provide a setting that is conducive to openness than a focus group (unless the group is carefully constructed with friends or peers as participants) and will be useful as your proposal's method of data collection. Key disadvantages are the extent to which the researcher can 'lead' or bias responses, participants can be intimidated, responses can be misinterpreted and participants may fail to turn up.

Recording the interview

It's by far the best practice to record interviews and this should be written into your proposal. Saying you'll use field notes that you write up after the interview will not give you the depth, immediacy or nuance that is required, and won't allow you to transcribe verbatim and quote participants. Recording interviews allows you to:

- give participants your full attention rather than dividing it between writing and listening;
- obtain a full record of the interview that you can make notes from and come back to; but your participant might be uncomfortable with recording or might be more wary of being open and honest.

The two options for recording your interviews are video or audio recording. Video recording captures non-verbal communication but is rarely used because it is so intrusive. Audio recording is generally regarded as good enough without being too disruptive. You can use either tape or digital audio recording.

Transcribing audio recording of interviews

Transcribing audio recordings of interviews is a time-consuming process. One hour of interview can take 2–6 hours to transcribe and the transcript from a one-hour interview can be 20–40 pages (Boyatzis, 1998). Although it may seem like just a boring administrative task, it is far more than that, and you need to acknowledge this in your proposal: analysis begins with basic listening to recordings to see patterns occurring. Transcribing provides a useful opportunity to continue this analysis before you begin the formal process of data analysis (see Chapter 5 for a detailed discussion of data analysis).

Researcher reflexivity

While quantitative research has traditionally used the concept of objectivity to seek to remove the researcher from the study through addressing issues of bias, qualitative research argues that this is neither possible nor necessarily desirable. In qualitative research, an alternative criterion for establishing trustworthiness is confirmability, which refers to the extent to which the data obtained from interviews are shaped by the participant rather than the personal interests, values and biases of the interviewer (Lincoln and Guba, 1985). This requires you to be aware of what you bring to the task of interviewing your participants at multiple levels. At a practical level, this involves you being aware of how you may inadvertently shape the responses of your participants, e.g. by nodding enthusiastically when participants provide responses that you agree with and having neutral or negative body language when they make statements that you disagree with. At a deeper level, it is about your own reflexivity as a researcher, which is central to qualitative research.

The concept of reflexivity acknowledges that we bring our own thoughts, values and beliefs derived from our personal and professional background to our research. Viewed from a reflexive point of view, subjectivity is not a problem but an asset. For example, our experiences may sensitise us to aspects of a situation that others would overlook. But we need to be conscious of how our experiences may also mean that we are unaware of, or make assumptions about, other aspects of the situation. It is not possible for us to be free from assumptions, but reflexivity enables us to become aware of and explicit about these assumptions. To illustrate this, see the case study below.

Case study: Researcher reflexivity

Susan is a nursing student who is interested in undertaking qualitative interviews with nursing staff in an emergency department about managing patients who have injuries related to drinking alcohol. As she is developing the proposal, she has been keeping a reflexive journal.

In a journal entry, she reflected upon her own experiences and attitudes towards alcohol and how these may have influenced her approach. She reflected upon how her family tended to drink on family occasions and how she enjoyed this. She also reflected upon the attitude she had towards drinking in her peer group both as she grew up and in her current student group, where drinking was an essential part of her social life. She explored how this had shaped her attitudes towards alcohol, including her interest in the research topic itself.

She become worried that she was not 'objective' and thought that another student from a different background, e.g. someone who had grown up in a family where drinking alcohol was not acceptable, might approach the topic from a more objective perspective.

Activity 4.3   *Researcher reflexivity*

1. How might Susan's background influence how she approaches interviews with participants?
2. To what extent do you think that the other student that she envisaged would be more objective?

There is a brief outline answer at the end of the chapter.

Ethical data management

The Data Protection Act (1998) means that researchers handling personal information must comply with various principles and gives participants rights over their personal information.

Your proposal will need to address these issues and some suggestions concerning how this might be achieved are as follows.

You must also comply with the Act in full, or make the data completely anonymous so that the data now fall outside the Act's definition of personal data. This will be the case when it is impossible to identify the individuals from their data. This includes any other information held. An anonymous list with a separate key listing participants by a number or pseudonym will still not be completely anonymous under the terms of the Act, so you must anonymise data and not keep a record of who is who in the study. In this case you can use the data without making arrangements to comply with the Data Protection Act because the data will no longer fall within the Act's definition of personal data (University of Plymouth, 2009).

You have a duty to ensure that participants' information is kept safe in a locked or otherwise secure location. Any papers must be kept in a locked filing cabinet and shredded when no longer required. Transcripts held as computer files should be password-protected so that the data are protected by a double layer of security: an initial password verification when logging in and a password for each individual folder or file. You can also encrypt data: this is even more secure. When deleting electronic data it is not enough simply to press delete and empty the recycle bin as this only removes the file name; the data will still be accessible to a knowledgeable third party. Instead data must be destroyed securely or 'shredded'. Software for password protecting and encrypting data is already loaded in Windows PCs and Apple Macs. For shredding folders and files, Microsoft has a tool that is free to download and Apple's is already built into Macs. The relevant websites giving details are at the end of the chapter. Memory sticks should be avoided as they are too easy to lose. Check how long you are required by your university to keep data. It may be as long as ten years after completion of the study.

Focus groups

This section introduces you to another commonly used research method that may inform your proposals: focus groups. Focus groups have entered the popular imagination following their controversial use in the early years of the New Labour government (Barbour and Kitzinger, 1999). Although group interviews have a long history in market research and were used to evaluate propaganda during the Second World War, it is only relatively recently that focus groups have become a popular and respected research method in the social sciences (Morgan, 1997). This can be contrasted with anthropological techniques, which have been around for over 100 years.

Focus groups are versatile and have been used for a wide range of topics. For example, focus groups have been used to research infertility in British South Asian communities (Culley et al., 2007), children's experiences of mental health services (Day et al., 2006), women's health in rural India (Vissandjée et al., 2002), female genital mutilation in Switzerland (Thierfelder et al., 2005) and access to out-of-hours health services by members of the Vietnamese community in London (Free et al., 1999).

Defining focus groups

A focus group is a group of individuals selected to provide their opinions on a defined subject, facilitated by a moderator who aims to create an open and relaxed environment and promote interaction between participants. Rather than an interview with a number of participants giving their views, focus groups enable discussion between participants (Kitzinger, 1994). Such discussions can enable participants to explore and challenge each other's views and can result in people clarifying and changing their views, and this interaction could be an important factor in deciding to choose them for your proposal.

Combining focus groups with other research methods

Focus groups are often used on their own, but can be combined with other research methods, such as surveys or interviews (Morgan, 1993, 1997). You may want to use focus groups before a survey to provide an overview and test the range of opinions, which will be used in questionnaire construction. For example, the Scottish Executive used focus groups to develop a national survey for people from minority ethnic communities (Scottish Executive, 2003).

Interviews can be used in conjunction with focus groups where participants may disclose more sensitive information than they would in a group setting. Whereas focus groups are effective in accessing shared public knowledge, interviews are fruitful for more personal, biographical information. For research topics that require both forms of knowledge, combining both methods can be productive.

Research summary: Combining focus groups and interviews

Michell (1999) conducted a longitudinal study of teenage lifestyles that followed a cohort of 11- and 12-year-olds over time. She sought to understand how changing peer group structures influenced health behaviours. She used a combination of focus groups and interviews to examine teenage relationships, particularly the 'pecking order' in peer relationships.

Michell found that there were three identifiable groups: 'top' or popular girls, 'middle' girls and marginalised or 'bottom' girls. One of the most interesting insights was the difference between the data revealed in the focus groups compared to the interviews. For 'top' and 'middle' girls, there was little difference between what they said in the focus groups and what they said in the interviews. For marginalised or 'bottom' girls, the picture was quite different. While 'top' and 'middle' girls acknowledged their own status in the focus groups, 'bottom' girls did not and were often quieter and sometimes silent. 'Bottom' girls only acknowledged their status in individual interviews and discussed their difficulties in school and often at home.

This difference was only noted in 'low-status' girls. By contrast, Michell found that 'low-status' boys responded in focus groups and interviews in similar ways. She described them as *either silent or at best monosyllabic in both settings or were silly and disruptive, relating wildly implausible anecdotes about violence and drug use, etc.* (Michell, 1999, page 46).

This interesting study provides a useful insight into the limitations of focus groups for topics that require subjects to discuss both public, shared knowledge and personal, biographical information. Combining both methods enabled the researcher to access both forms of knowledge successfully.

Advantages and disadvantages of focus groups

Focus groups enable you to gain a range of opinions about a topic in a fairly easy and reliable way. They can produce significant amounts of data focused on a specific topic and are less time-consuming than interviews. They provide an opportunity for participants to express a range of opinions and challenge and interact with one another in an open environment. Participants can explore and develop their opinions through interactions with others and provide insights into complex behaviours. They are often seen as more democratic in that there may be six or eight participants but only one researcher, who is therefore 'outnumbered', and the power differential between researcher and participants is less than in a one-to-one setting. Finally, they are more accessible than other research methods for people with literacy difficulties (Owen, 2001) or for people who do not have English as a first language (Barbour and Kitzinger, 1999).

Arranging times and venues for a group of people to meet can be complex and demanding, however, and require you to engage in considerable negotiation and coordination. Some group members may feel unable to voice their opinions because they feel less confident or less powerful or feel their opinions may be unacceptable to other group members. Recruiting group members from similar backgrounds and a skilled moderator can significantly reduce these risks. The nature of the group context may mean participants do not discuss personal experiences and histories in as much depth or detail as individual interviews (Morgan, 1997; Michell, 1999). Recording and transcribing can be time-consuming and complex; for example, identifying the contribution of different participants from an audio tape when they have similar voices. Finally, focus groups offer less control over the discussion than an interview.

When not to use focus groups

There are a number of circumstances when focus groups are best avoided, and you need to think these through carefully before proposing them in your project. First, when boundary issues may become too complex; for example, participants have complex relationships with each other that involve potential role conflicts. Second, when you are seeking to learn about the individual history and biography of participants (Morgan, 1997; Michell, 1999). Third, when you are seeking to make statistical generalisations about a wider population. Fourth, where it would be extremely difficult to bring participants together at a certain time and venue. Finally, if you are relatively new to research, avoid using focus groups to discuss issues that are likely to be very distressing to participants. Focus groups have been successfully used for sensitive topics (Zeller, 1993; Farquhar with Das, 1999), but require considerable experience and skills in moderation, although don't let this put you off planning them in your work.

Selection and recruitment issues

There is considerable debate about the 'ideal' size for a focus group. Although groups of 8–12 are thought desirable for market research purposes, social research usually uses smaller group sizes, often 6–8 participants (Barbour and Kitzinger, 1999; Krueger and Casey, 2000). It can also depend upon how aware the participants are of the topic – larger groups are necessary when participants have low levels of awareness, whereas smaller groups enable highly aware participants to discuss the topic in detail (Morgan, 1997). Drop out (usually 10–20%) occurs, and must be planned for.

When deciding how many focus groups to plan, the general consensus for large-scale projects is that it is best to plan three or four focus groups with any one type of participant, that is, three different groups of nurses (Morgan, 1997, 1998; Krueger and Casey, 2000).

Student research proposals often plan one or two focus groups. Different university supervisors or tutors will have different opinions on this, but 1–3 groups usually provide sufficient useful and stimulating data to analyse.

'Naturally occurring' and 'stranger' groups

There are two types of focus group: a 'naturally occurring' group and a 'stranger' group. The naturally occurring group comprises participants who know each other in another role, such as a work team or support group. The stranger or assembled group comprises people who do not know each other but have a similar background or similar experiences. Neither is regarded as being 'better' than the other and your choice depends upon your research proposal.

A potential issue when using naturally occurring groups is the possibility of 'groupthink', although this can occur in any group. This is the tendency for dissenters in groups to suppress their opinions and for the group to reach a consensus quickly without critically considering the alternatives to avoid conflict (Janis, 1982; Morgan, 1997). This can be challenged and explored by a sensitive moderator and can lead to rich and interesting data.

If your research focuses on the 'taken for granted' assumptions underlying a topic, a stranger group may have the advantage that participants are likely to spend more time explaining their reasoning (Morgan, 1998). Stranger groups are popular in market research for this reason, whereas naturally occurring groups are more common in student research.

Recruiting and selecting participants

You need to outline your recruitment strategy in your proposal. Participants for a natural group can be recruited in a number of ways. One of the easiest ways is to use existing networks; for example, designing a poster or e-mail to be distributed, being invited to meetings to explain your research. Asking a key figure to distribute information can be effective, provided participants do not feel under pressure to participate. Some research projects offer incentives, such as gift tokens, but providing refreshments and food can be equally successful.

In your plan, you should aim to minimise recruitment bias rather than achieve generalisability (Curtis and Redmond, 2007). Recruitment bias occurs when groups do not reflect the diversity of potential participants. For example, planning a focus group evaluating a service by approaching the manager for details of potential participants is likely to generate a list of service users who feel positively about the service. It is difficult to eliminate this entirely; for example, a poster invitation will still attract people who normally get involved in such activities. Any method has strengths and weaknesses and these must be acknowledged in proposals. If you are seeking to be able to generalise statistical findings to a much wider population, a quantitative approach such as surveys with a larger sample size using the relevant statistical tests is necessary.

Homogeneous or heterogeneous group?

Although there is debate whether focus groups should be homogeneous (similar) or heterogeneous (dissimilar), most researchers prefer a homogeneous group who share a background or experiences that are the focus of the discussion (Vaughn et al., 1996; Morgan, 1998). Having a homogeneous group is advantageous because it can help to ensure that participants feel able to speak freely and lead to data that are more straightforward to analyse (Krueger and Casey, 2000). Heterogeneous groups are particularly problematic where there are power differentials between participants because apparent consensus may not reflect the real views of all members (Krueger and Casey, 2000; Happel, 2007).

If participants are selected to be placed in groups of similar people, known as 'segmenting', the most common categories in large-scale research projects are gender, race, age and social class (Morgan, 1997). For nursing students, the categories are more likely to be related to role or grades within particular roles – for example, service users or patients, critical care nurses, Band 5 and 6 nurses, healthcare assistants and assistant practitioners and so on – though the previously mentioned factors should also be considered where relevant.

> ### Case study: Planning a focus group
>
> *David is on placement in a large, acute-sector NHS hospital trust. He is interested in nurses' views on improving patient care in a coronary care unit.*
>
> *David decided that a focus group would be a good research method because it would enable him to hear a range of views and for participants to interact with each other and challenge each other's views. His focus was on participants' professional experience rather than their personal biographies and it would take much longer to conduct interviews that would produce a similar amount of data. The disadvantages are that it can be difficult to arrange for a group of people to meet, the risk of 'groupthink' and the possibility that some group members do not feel able to express their opinions.*
>
> *David considered how to select his participants and how many focus groups to run. There are 50 full- and part-time nurses in the team, a senior matron and her three deputy managers. Sixteen staff members were interested in being involved and David decided against involving the manager and deputies because the power differential might make it difficult for participants to speak openly. He decided to run two focus groups, with qualified nurses in one group and unqualified ones in the other, to gain perspectives from the different staff groups and to prevent the unqualified staff from feeling inhibited by their 'seniors'.*

Discussion guides

A discussion guide is a list of topics or questions that you produce for yourself as the moderator to guide the conversation in a focus group. It is likely that you'll need to include this in your proposal. Assuming a two-hour focus group, it is realistic to ask 8–12 questions, depending upon the type of question (Krueger and Casey, 2000). The group nature of the discussions means that fewer questions are asked than in individual interviews.

A discussion guide should have a clear structure and will include a range of different types of question:

1. Introduction: summarises the research topic briefly, confidentiality, recording and ground rules. Morgan (1997) suggests:

    *   only one person speaking at a time;
    *   no side conversations among neighbours;
    *   everyone participating, with no one dominating;
    *   keep it as brief as possible.

2. Warm-up questions: these aim to help participants feel comfortable with speaking in the group and are usually short, factual questions that every participant responds to. Ensuring that everyone makes an initial statement can also reduce the risk of groupthink (Morgan, 1997).

3. Introductory questions: these introduce the topic and provide a context, encouraging participants to think about the key topics.

4. Key questions: these are the principal questions that directly address your research question. Up to half of the questions will be in this category.
5. Closing questions: these enable the moderator to check his or her understanding of what has been said, to enable participants to provide a summary view and to provide an opportunity for any issues not discussed to be addressed. Krueger and Casey (2000) identify three questions in this category:

- The 'all-things-considered' question: used to clarify the final position of participants on the topics discussed and their relative importance (e.g. 'all things considered, what is the most important issue we have discussed here today?'). This is particularly important if participants have changed their views and if they have discussed relatively minor issues more frequently than more important issues.
- The summary question: the moderator attempts to summarise the discussion and asks whether it is a fair synopsis.
- The final question: having summarised the discussion, the moderator asks whether anything has been overlooked or whether participants want to add anything that they haven't previously said. Ask this with ten minutes left rather than at the very end, when participants may want to finish on time.

Morgan (1997) uses the analogy of a funnel to describe the process of each focus group, starting with a less structured general discussion leading to a more structured discussion of specific topics. This allows the first part of the group to concentrate on participants' own perspectives on the topic and the second part to focus on the interviewer's specific interests in the topic (Morgan, 1997).

Organising pilot focus groups is more difficult than pilot interviews, but you can get feedback that can significantly improve a discussion guide. The two best stages to involve other people are the initial stage of generating possible questions and the final stage of developing your discussion guide.

Case study: Developing a discussion guide

David developed his discussion guide by involving his practice mentor and a staff member from another team to generate some ideas for questions. Using a flipchart and pen, they spent 30 minutes generating as many questions as possible. He took these questions away and redrafted them, ensuring they were in the right sequence. He took them back to his practice assessor and colleague and they provided useful feedback.

It is unlikely that you'll need to say much about the role of the group moderator in a proposal, but the moderator's function is:

- to create an open and relaxed environment and promote interaction between participants;
- to promote the involvement of all participants without allowing particular individuals to dominate.

Having a colleague or fellow student who can assist you is essential and this should be acknowledged in your proposal resources. As well as helping you to welcome participants and other practical support, they can take field notes, as it is virtually impossible to moderate well and take notes simultaneously. A debriefing session will help to clarify your ideas after the group's end.

It is unlikely that you'll need to say much about managing the group in a proposal, but key points are:

- a focus group is not a therapy or support group;
- its purpose is to gather data for your research project;
- try not to let groups become side-tracked with issues that are important to them but are not relevant to the research.

Case study: David's focus group

It is the day of David's first focus group and one person is off ill and another can't get away from the unit. This still leaves six people and David has decided to go ahead. A colleague has agreed to act as assistant moderator, taking notes.

The group starts well, with participants writing down and then discussing their first impressions of the issues. When David asks them about improving patient care, one participant states the whole team is already overworked, particularly as there is an unfilled vacancy. There is general unrest in the group and one participant starts whispering to another. The conversation turns to feeling overworked and undervalued in the service.

Activity 4.4   *Reflection*

If you were David, how would you respond to this situation in your role as moderator?

There is a brief outline answer at the end of the chapter.

Recording and transcribing

Video recording would be ideal from a data-gathering perspective, but is likely to be too intrusive for participants and the equipment is unlikely to be available. Audio recording is the most common compromise, enabling a recording to be kept while not being too intrusive.

Krueger (1994) identifies a range of choices when writing up recordings, depending upon the rigour of your analysis and the time you have available:

- A full transcript: a verbatim transcript is produced and used alongside notes taken during the focus group and afterwards. For some forms of analysis (e.g. conversational analysis), transcripts should include every aspect of the conversation, including pauses and all verbal communication.

- Tape-based analysis and shortened transcript: a transcript is produced, but it covers the points made rather than being a verbatim account.
- Note-based analysis: this relies mainly on notes, a debriefing session and summary comments made at the end of the focus group. The session is taped but the tape is used to verify specific quotes.
- Memory-based analysis: notes can be consulted but most of the write-up is based upon recall.

Best practice is to fully transcribe the tape recordings and you should propose this in your plan. However, it may be acceptable to propose a lesser arrangement if focus groups are planned as a preliminary or exploratory measure for other research methods, such as surveys (Curtis and Redmond, 2007).

Chapter summary

This chapter has introduced you to the key features of interviews as a research method. You have considered when it would be most appropriate to use interviews compared to alternative approaches such as questionnaires and focus group analysis. After studying the different types of interview, you examined some of the key issues around recruiting and selecting participants and applied this to a student case study.

This chapter has also looked at how to develop an interview schedule and understand the range of interview questions that are available to you. You reviewed the functions of different types of question, paying particular attention to questions to avoid. A learning point from this chapter has been the importance of preparation, as careful thought at the early stages can save valuable time in the later stages.

Despite the challenges involved, interviewing is a popular and rewarding research method. It enables you to gain rich and complex data about people's knowledge, experiences, views and attitudes. You have seen in this chapter that careful preparation can avoid the common pitfalls and help you to produce a research project that is well designed, interesting and useful.

Focus groups are an increasingly popular research method that has been used to study a wide range of issues. They can be used as a stand-alone method or combined with other research methods, such as interviews or surveys.

Focus groups have a range of advantages and disadvantages. They enable you to gain a range of opinions in a fairly easy and reliable way and can produce significant amounts of data focused on a specific topic. They are less time-consuming than interviews and are more accessible than other research methods for people with literacy difficulties, people whose first language is not English and for traditionally marginalised groups.

(continued)

continued … •

However, they can be difficult to arrange and recording and transcribing can be complex and time-consuming.

Focus groups can be either naturally occurring groups or stranger groups. Each has its strengths and weaknesses and neither is inherently better. Focus groups in social research tend to be smaller than in market research, often involving 6–8 participants. While large-scale studies involve three or more focus groups per category of participant to exhaust a topic, student research commonly involves one or two groups.

Different methods of recording focus groups were examined.

Activity answers

Activity 4.1: Critical thinking (page 69)

Victoria does not need to use convenience or snowball sampling because she has a number of potential participants who she can contact relatively easily. Since she is not using grounded theory to analyse her data, theoretical sampling is not necessary and quota sampling is rarely used in academic research, except in grounded theory. The most appropriate sampling strategy would be purposive sampling, in which she selects participants who are most likely to yield useful information. This is often based upon factors such as the participant's knowledge, experience or role. She decided to interview two groups of voluntary sector staff, one working in her placement agency and another in a similar voluntary organisation in a neighbouring area. She will focus on staff members who are likely to experience partnership working as part of their everyday role.

Activity 4.2: Decision making (page 70)

1. Construct a research question for her: 'How do voluntary sector mental health staff view partnership working with statutory organisations?'
2. Think of five questions which she might ask workers that would support that research question by allowing participants to talk about the issue and give her relevant data. Examples might include the following:

    *   Tell me a bit about your relationship with staff in the statutory sector.
    *   Tell me a bit about your relationship with organisations in the statutory sector.
    *   What are the good things about working with the statutory sector?
    *   What are the bad things about working with the statutory sector?
    *   How could you and your organisation improve your working relationships with the statutory sector?

3. The initial four questions are essential and the last desirable, as the research question is about how voluntary sector mental health staff view partnership working with statutory organisations rather than changing that relationship.

Activity 4.3: Researcher reflexivity (page 73)

1. When Susan interviews participants, she may find that she inadvertently agrees slightly too enthusiastically when participants take an 'alcohol isn't that bad, we all do it' attitude while she

is silent or appears disapproving when participants criticise patients for drinking any alcohol at all.

2. From the perspective of reflexivity in qualitative research, neither student would be 'objective'. Each would simply bring different experiences, values and beliefs to the research topic. Rather than seeking to attain perfect 'objectivity', the aim of reflexivity is for researchers both to be aware of what they bring and to be open and explicit about this in the research process.

Activity 4.4: Reflection (page 80)

The risk is that the discussion is likely to get side-tracked into a general discussion about staff shortages and the additional work pressures this causes. While this is important to the team, it is not productive for the research question.

If participants become side-tracked with an issue that they feel is important for them but which is tangential to your topic, you need to bring them back to the research questions. It is important to do this sensitively so participants do not feel censured. For example, you could say 'That's an important topic, but I would like to hear more about . . .'. If participants continue, it is important to persist; for example, saying 'perhaps we can come back to that later, but X made an interesting point and I would like to hear more about . . .'.

When groups get side-tracked by other issues, one thing to consider is whether the question is quite difficult or challenging for participants and they are avoiding responding to it. If the group continues to get side-tracked, it can be helpful to ask directly whether the question is difficult to respond to. Expressing this openly enables participants either to address the question directly or to explore the reasons why it might be a difficult topic to talk about. Either way, it will produce useful data that are relevant to the research question.

Further reading

On interviews

Kvale, S and Brinkmann, S (2009) *InterViews: Learning the Craft of Qualitative Research Interviewing*, 2nd edition. London: Sage.
The second edition of a classic text on interviews, which places interviewing firmly within the qualitative tradition. Chapter 7 provides a practical overview of the interview process, while the early chapters address key theoretical issues.

Mason, J (2002) *Qualitative Researching*, 2nd edition. London: Sage.
A solid and well-written textbook that combines practical considerations with detailed consideration of theoretical and methodological issues. Chapter 4 on qualitative interviewing is particularly clear and helpful.

On focus groups

Barbour, RS and Kitzinger, J (1999) *Developing Focus Group Research: Politics, Theory and Practice.* London: Sage.
Excellent edited collection discussing specific issues about the use of focus groups.

Krueger, RA and Casey, MA (2000) *Focus Groups*, 3rd edition. California: Sage.
An excellent introductory text giving sound, practical advice.

Morgan, DL (1997) *Focus Groups as Qualitative Research*, 2nd edition. London: Sage.
Another good introductory text, quite short but covers the major topics.

Sim, J (1998) Collecting and analysing qualitative data: issues raised by the focus group. *Journal of Advanced Nursing*, 28 (2): 345–352.
A helpful article about data analysis issues for focus groups.

Useful websites

www.opsi.gov.uk/Acts/Acts1998/ukpga_19980029_en_1
The Data Protection Act (1998). Researchers should familiarise themselves with Part 1 and Schedules 1, 2 and 3 of the Act.

Protecting folders and files

For Microsoft PCs, see: **http://office.microsoft.com**
For Apple Macs, see: **www.macworld.com**

Shredding

For Microsoft PCs, see: **http://technet.microsoft.com/en-us/sysinternals/bb897443.aspx** for a free tool to download.
For Apple Macs, see: **www.macworld.com**

Chapter 5
Analysing qualitative data

Chapter aims

After reading this chapter, you should be able to:

- understand the concept of thematic analysis of qualitative data;
- use thematic analysis to inform strategies for planning a proposal;
- be aware of the particular issues that apply to data gathered from focus group discussions;
- use your understanding of data analysis to critique qualitative research findings.

Introduction

In this chapter, we look at approaches to data analysis, examining the analysis of data from interviews and focus groups. We will start from the perspective of choosing potential strategies when planning a proposal and will make reference to aspects that are important when critiquing research findings.

Data analysis is the process that researchers use to make sense of the information collected and in searching for what lies below the surface content in order to grasp how to understand the often complex story that their data tell. Qualitative data analysis can be likened to skills that we use every day in our nursing practice: when we meet a new patient or client, we seek to understand that person's unique situation. When we have met a number of them in similar situations, we start to see patterns in what they tell us. We try to identify similarities and differences and start to see links and relationships between the different aspects of their experiences. This helps us to build up our understanding of those experiences that can be helpful for new service users that we meet.

Qualitative data analysis also involves new skills and techniques, which can seem daunting and confusing at first: it is not helpful to see it as a highly technical, almost mystical process, but neither is it true that findings will be obvious in the mass of data collected. Developing themes and writing these in a coherent manner which addresses the aims and objectives of a study is in itself a skill, which can be developed and is best understood in the context of existing methods which give an element of structure and robustness to the analysis.

Analysing qualitative data

The term 'data analysis' may provoke images of number crunching and statistical tests. However, in qualitative research, the data being analysed are words. These are the words of participants during interviews and focus groups. It is possible to analyse visual material or observational data, but these are specialised areas not covered in this book. In qualitative research, data analysis is the fascinating process of making sense of what people have said, identifying patterns and understanding meanings. Miles and Huberman (1994) capture the inherently interesting nature of this process:

> *Qualitative data are sexy. They are a source of well-grounded, rich descriptions and explanations of processes in identifiable local contexts. With qualitative data one can preserve chronological flow, see precisely which events led to which consequences, and derive fruitful explanations.*
> (Miles and Huberman, 1994, page 1)

While you have to be consistent and systematic in how you interpret your data, the complexity of how to interpret meaning means that rigid rules for data analysis are rarely possible or indeed helpful. Qualitative data analysis is a contested area, with no universally agreed rules and many different interpretations in a variety of authoritative textbooks. There are, however, broad guidelines and applying them requires researchers to exercise judgement and make explicit decisions. This section will concentrate upon data collected from interviews and focus groups.

Alternative approaches to analysing qualitative data

There are a wide range of approaches to analysing qualitative data to choose from, coming from different research traditions. It is important to choose an approach to data analysis that is compatible with your research question and overall research approach. Some methods of data analysis require you to adopt a specific research approach, such as grounded theory and interpretative phenomenological analysis (IPA), while others are compatible with a wide range of research approaches, such as thematic analysis. In this chapter, grounded theory and thematic analysis will be discussed as two of the most common approaches. Grounded theory will be briefly outlined but the primary focus will be on thematic analysis as a sound and robust approach for new researchers.

Grounded theory was developed in the late 1960s as qualitative data analysis was becoming more widely accepted (Glaser and Strauss, 1967). It was developed as a systematic way of analysing data that seeks to address concerns at that time that qualitative research did not meet the standards of validity and reliability expected in quantitative research. Grounded theory is an approach to research that emphasises the importance of generating new concepts and theoretical frameworks from data. The name 'grounded theory' captures its aim of seeking to generate theory that is grounded in the careful analysis of data, rather than the testing of existing theory. There are different schools within grounded theory, starting with Glaser and Strauss (1967) developing different versions of grounded theory after their original publication, and no single version predominates.

Grounded theory is not just a method for analysing data but a whole approach to research. Key concepts in grounded theory are constant comparison, theoretical sampling and theoretical saturation. Data collection and analysis happen alongside one another and data are analysed as they are collected in a continuous process of constant comparison. Theoretical sampling is an approach in which sampling evolves as the research develops rather than being predetermined. For example, early data collection and analysis in an observational study about dignity on hospital wards may suggest that 'privacy' is an important category so the researcher can seek opportunities to observe settings where patient privacy is central. Early sampling is usually directed towards having a wide variety of data, which is progressively narrowed as the analysis develops. This continues until new data do not provide any new insights, the point known as theoretical saturation.

Grounded theory has been subjected to a number of criticisms. The claims by grounded theory that it generates theory have been disputed. It is argued that, in many instances, what is generated are findings that are specific to particular localised settings rather than formal theory, though they may have wider applicability. Grounded theory discourages researchers from conducting extensive literature reviews before starting data collection because this can lead to findings that are grounded more in the existing literature rather than the data. However, the ability of researchers to suspend their existing knowledge until the later stages of analysis has been questioned more recently and it is now generally accepted that theory-free observation is unrealistic (Bryman, 2012).

Understanding thematic analysis

Although you will find other methods, a very common model for analysing qualitative data is *thematic analysis* (Davies, 2007; Bryman, 2012). We will introduce you to this clear and systematic way of analysing your data based upon a model of thematic analysis developed by Braun and Clarke (2006).

Thematic analysis has been defined as *a method for identifying, analysing and reporting patterns (themes) within data* (Braun and Clarke, 2006, page 79). It is a foundational method that offers core skills that are useful for other forms of qualitative analysis. Thematic analysis is a flexible approach that is compatible with different epistemological approaches. We have previously discussed the distinction between positivist/realist and interpretivist/social constructionist approaches (see Chapter 1) and thematic analysis can be used with both approaches.

The process of thematic analysis

Braun and Clarke (2006) outline a six-stage model for the process of analysing data. Before we look at this in detail, it is important to define some key terms. Data set refers to the total data collected that will be used in the analysis. Data item refers to a particular interview or focus group, while data extract refers to a passage that has been taken from a data item such as a quote from an interview. Research reports should contain some information about the processes used to analyse data and the information below will help you to understand what they should have done and therefore identify any potential critique of their methods.

Phase 1: Becoming familiar with the data

Data analysis should begin with the immersion of the researchers in the data by reading through all the transcripts at least once, which will enable them to become sensitised to the material and develop an awareness of the whole data set. Where one researcher has collected and transcribed the data him/herself, he/she will already have a good level of prior knowledge of the key issues in the data set but seeing it written down can enable the person to see new patterns, particularly recurring words or phrases, or similar concepts which may be expressed slightly differently between data items and participants but have some commonality. This can be time-consuming and it can be tempting to skip it, but it will be time well spent. If more than one researcher is involved, each one will need to go through this process before moving on to the next steps.

Phase 2: Creating initial codes

Once researchers have familiarised themselves with the data, the next step is to generate the initial codes. A code is the most basic building block of data analysis and identifies a feature of the data that is of interest to the researcher (Boyatzis, 1998; Braun and Clarke, 2006). The example in the case study illustrates this process.

Case study: Coding interview transcripts

Emmanuel is a researcher who has been asked by a children's hospital to investigate how high-profile child deaths affect nursing staff in children's services. He interviewed a number of front-line children's nurses. Having reread his interview transcripts thoroughly, Emmanuel started coding his first transcript and began with the following passage from a children's nurse (Figure 5.1).

Transcript	Codes
Interviewer: *How does a high-profile child death affect you as a children's nurse?* Participant 1: *It creates a lot more anxiety in front-line nurses, definitely. And it's hard to deal with that anxiety when you get so little clinical supervision. So you tend to find ways to cope with it, some positive and some negative. The positive ways are that I tend to go out of my way to document everything in the smallest detail and make sure I've got my paperwork constantly up to date. The negative ways are that this means that I work even longer hours, as I can't do all the paperwork during a normal shift so I have to stay behind and get off late, and so I get more tired, so it's more likely I'll make a mistake.*	'A lot more anxiety' 'Little supervision' 'Positive ways of coping' 'Negative ways of coping'

Figure 5.1: Interview transcript

Comment

As you can see, the transcript is divided into two columns. In the first column are the words of the participants, while the second column is left blank for Emmanuel's codes. The transcript should be double-line-spaced and it can be helpful to number the lines for ease of reference.

Reflecting the participant's words

In the example shown in the case study, Emmanuel has decided that the best way to reflect the participant's words is to reproduce them faithfully. Technically, this is known as *emic* or 'in vivo' coding because it relates to the words and phrases used by participants. The alternative approach is *etic* or analytical codes, which are devised by the researcher and usually relate to the theoretical perspective that underpins the analysis. For example, if the same data were analysed using a psychoanalytic framework, the coding for 'ways of coping' might be termed 'defence mechanisms'.

The process of coding data involves breaking it down into its smallest parts (codes) before rebuilding it into major patterns (themes). To use a metaphor, imagine the transcript is made up of children's coloured bricks. When researchers are coding data, they are breaking down what participants have said into its smallest constituent parts (bricks) and deciding what colour each part should be. For example, participants talked about 'negative ways of coping' during the interview: each example of this can be coded and given a particular colour (e.g. red). All of the 'red bricks' (data extracts coded as red) within the interview and across all of the interviews can be gathered together.

The metaphor has its limitations because it suggests that the coloured building bricks are already contained in the data and jump out with minimal effort, whereas in reality this is a complex process that can take many iterations before the 'colours' become evident. It may be tempting to think of data analysis as being a passive process of themes 'emerging' from interview or focus group transcripts, but it needs to be a much more active and scholarly event which can take days.

'Emerging codes or themes' can, at one level, be a reassuring image because it presents the view that knowledge exists out there to be discovered and implies that data analysis is an objective, scientific process in which the analyst has an objective role. For experienced researchers this is not a sustainable view as data analysis is an active process in which choices are continually made and to which they bring their previous experience and the experience of interviewing participants. Some might regard these as 'contaminants' or 'biases' that should be removed in order to obtain an 'objective' view, but in qualitative research, removing the self and personal experiences from the research process is neither possible nor desirable. Instead, it is about being reflexive – about questioning personal assumptions and views and being open about them in data analysis and subsequent write-ups.

What is important is that equal attention is given, as material that may seem unpromising initially may become important later. Although this will rarely be discussed in research reports, a large number of codes will initially be developed and this will allow researchers to generate potential themes while also retaining some of the surrounding data to help to understand the context. Some sections of transcripts may not be coded because there is discussion or explanation of a concept in some detail, while other sections may receive more than one code if many concepts are being outlined: *You can code individual extracts in as many different 'themes' as they fit into – so an extract may be uncoded, coded once, or coded many times, as relevant* (Braun and Clarke, 2006, page 89).

Once the transcripts are coded and there are data extracts relating to a particular code, these are grouped together with some identifying information for ease of analysis when building themes. For example, see the case study below.

> ### Case study: Theming topics
>
> *As Emmanuel undertakes further interviews, he will add any further mention of 'negative ways of coping'. At the end of the process, he will have a file called 'negative ways of coping' that will contain all of the participants' words when they were discussing this topic (Table 5.1).*

Code: 'negative ways of coping'
Participant 1
The negative ways are that this means that I work even longer hours, as I can't do all the paperwork during a normal shift so I have to stay behind and get off late, and so I get more tired, so it's more likely I'll make a mistake. Line 22
Participant 2
I find that a high-profile child death can have a negative effect because I tend to cope with it by going to my manager all the time for every minor decision because I feel less anxious if I share the responsibility. Line 44
Participant 3
I find that, after a high-profile child death, I document everything very carefully and defensively. Rather than writing your notes and thinking 'how would this look if the parents read it?', you start thinking 'how would this look if it was read out at any inquiry panel?' (Pause) It's quite frightening really, I try not to think about it. Line 72

Table 5.1: Coded extracts

This is time-consuming when done properly but is an essential step; the raw transcripts containing thousands of words are being sifted and the building blocks of data analysis are being put together to inform and give coherent themes.

By the end of this stage, there will be a large number of codes along with their related data extracts. In the next stage, themes will be identified, which means seeing which of the 'colours' seem to link together (e.g. red bricks with pink and orange bricks). These wider groupings are called themes and there are likely to be a much smaller number of them.

Phase 3: Searching for themes

When a list of the codes has been produced, the next phase is to group them into potential themes. In this phase, the researchers' aim is to see how the codes can be grouped together into broader themes and how these themes relate to each other. Using the analogy of the coloured bricks, the transcripts have already been broken down into their constituent bricks but now the bricks are being grouped into collections of similar or compatible colours (e.g. red bricks being grouped with pink and orange bricks).

So what are themes? Themes are broader than codes and represent a higher level of abstraction. A theme *captures something important about the data in relation to the research question, and represents some level of patterned response or meaning within the data set* (Braun and Clarke, 2006, page 82). There are no rigid rules because we are dealing with the complexities of meaning, so researchers need to use their judgement. If more than one researcher is involved, they will need to resolve any disagreement by discussion until consensus is reached and their agreement is a step which adds rigour to the analysis as it demonstrates that the themes generated are not just the views of one person. This must all be done transparently and consistently. While the frequency with which a topic arises in the transcript is likely to be significant, there are no hard and fast rules. For example a rule like: 'if the theme occurs in more than 50% of the interview or focus group transcripts, it is a theme' is not helpful (Braun and Clarke, 2006), and there is an argument that qualitative researchers should avoid attempts at quantification in their data analysis.

Themes will frequently have more than one concept in them, and thus themes will be the overarching concepts while subthemes are similar or related issues. For example, Emmanuel has a theme of 'ways of coping', which has two subthemes: negative and positive ways of coping. Themes may have a clear relationship with each other; for example, whether the themes of 'ways of coping' and 'lack of supervision' are linked with the theme of 'increased anxiety of practitioners'.

As analysis progresses, some themes may become more important, while others become peripheral. Themes become more important because they say something significant about the research question or topic. Some codes do not fit into any group and can be grouped into a theme called 'miscellaneous', possibly on a temporary basis (Braun and Clarke, 2006). Eventually researchers may find they do not use all these 'miscellaneous' codes and can discard some of them.

At the end of this phrase, researchers will have developed a number of initial or candidate themes and subthemes that can be organised into an initial thematic map (Figure 5.2).

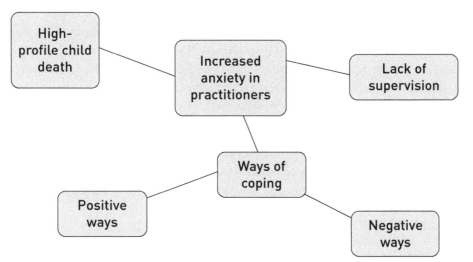

Figure 5.2: Thematic map

Phase 4: Reviewing themes

Having drawn up a list of potential or candidate themes and developed an initial thematic map, this phase focuses on reviewing and refining these themes. Data analysis, like so much of the research process, involves going back and forth between different stages in a recursive process.

In this phase, themes are reviewed at two levels. The first level is within the theme, in which all of the extracts from the transcripts are coded within that theme. As data extracts from each theme are examined, researchers will be evaluating critically whether the theme has sufficient data and whether they are sufficiently similar. If some themes have insufficient data or the data are too dissimilar then they are not sustainable themes. It may also be the case that what initially appears to be one theme needs to be split into two when the data are more carefully considered. Alternatively, your two initial themes may eventually prove to form one larger theme.

Within each theme, the data should clearly relate to it and be distinct from other themes. *Data within themes should cohere together meaningfully, whilst there should be clear and identifiable distinctions between themes* (Braun and Clarke, 2006, page 91).

Having reviewed codes within themes, the second level is to review across all of the transcripts. Here, researchers will review the themes overall to check that they reflect the meanings apparent in the total data set by standing back from the detailed reading of extracts to check whether the themes accurately reflect what participants said.

This all sounds easy! In fact, this is a complex but necessary step in the analysis as one frequent problem, particularly for novice researchers, is that they can end up with a lot of similar or closely related material spread across several themes, which could 'collapse down' into one major, overarching theme. This would simplify the analysis and make the write-up more convincing and coherent. Reading and rereading the themes and codes can help to overcome this; often this level of understanding develops over several days of work.

Phase 5: Defining and naming themes

Having developed a suitable thematic map, the next task is to define and refine the themes and to identify names that capture the core of what the theme is about. This requires a review of the data extracts upon which it was based. Rather than just paraphrasing the verbatim content, the key features of interest must be identified, probably in relation to your research aims and objectives or the broad area of interest. Within some themes, subthemes are likely to be present which organise the material. These need to be named too, and these names may contribute to naming the overarching themes in which they sit.

By the end of this stage, there will be a clear idea about what is included and what is not included in each theme; this will be achieved when each theme is clear, can be described in a couple of sentences and has names that are succinct and convey a coherent sense of what the theme is about.

Phase 6: Producing the report

In research reports, each theme should receive a detailed analysis, including how it fits into the overall narrative about the data. This stage begins when researchers have decided on a final set of themes and a thematic map. Writing up will be discussed in detail in Section 4.

Qualitative data analysis software

Qualitative data analysis (QDA) software is an alternative to coding data manually. Packages such as NVivo, AtlasTi, MaxQDA and the Ethnograph can separate out data extracts according to the codes assigned to them and help map out how they relate to each other. These software packages are quite expensive and are purchased by universities and by researchers as part of the grants and contracts they receive. It is necessary to have specialist training in how they work and, while in experienced hands they can be useful, the software does not actually do the analysis; it simply makes a researcher's own analysis easier as a process. See Gibbs (2007) and the two websites identified at the end of the chapter for discussion of different software packages.

Focus group data analysis issues

Focus group data analysis can proceed using the same processes as the thematic analysis derived from Braun and Clarke (2006), described above. However, although this may sound obvious, the purpose of a focus group is to represent the views of a group and their analysis thus has certain considerations that are different from when individuals are being interviewed separately. Most important of these is that participants in groups interact, discuss, challenge, clarify and generally engage in a dialogue rather than simply answer questions, and this interaction needs to be considered (Bloor et al., 2001) and should be reflected in data analysis processes and in research reports. This is frequently not clear when reading research reports but is important as it can add richness by reflecting diverse viewpoints in a group and show that researchers have acknowledged this and have taken it into account rather than simply picking quotes to support their own biases. The example in the case study illustrates this.

Case study: Data from focus group discussions

Emmanuel conducted a focus group to discuss how managers at the children's hospital react to high-profile child deaths in their management practices and support of children's nurses:

> *P1: What I tend to do is worry about it a lot in case there are any cases going on regarding children in our care which might be spotted by my nursing staff on the ward; this really gets to me when there is a high-profile case in the news as I dread something like Baby P happening here.*

Comment

This is giving only one manager's perspective, and although it is a clear example of her anxiety (which reflects what the nurses said in Emmanuel's individual interviews), it in no way reflects the views of the group. See how the picture is altered if an exchange of views is represented:

> *P1: What I tend to do is worry about it a lot in case there are any cases going on regarding children in our care which might be spotted by my nursing staff on the ward; this really gets to me when there is a high-profile case in the news as I dread something like Baby P happening here.*
>
> *P2: I dread it too – we all do, but let's not forget that we have invested a great deal of time and effort into establishing effective policies and procedures for safeguarding children in this directorate, and we have to have faith that these are appropriate and work as we intended.*
>
> *P3: Look, we now have in place compulsory, yearly training for all staff on this issue. I know we can't afford to be complacent and it would be awful if something did happen, but I do the training with them and I say it again and again, you must report anything suspicious. I give them the name and phone number of the safeguarding lead on a card so that they can phone her direct . . . we can't be everywhere at once as a team and we have to trust our staff to act appropriately.*
>
> *P4: I agree but it's still a huge worry.*
>
> *P1: Yes you're right but I still get sleepless nights about it sometimes.*
>
> *Having included an exchange of views on the issue rather than one simple quote, it is clear now that each participant in this manager's focus group has a significant level of anxiety about issues concerning safeguarding children, but the contextual information about the Trust's response is important and helps to offset the personal anxiety as they all know that appropriate policies and procedures are in place to help staff to respond. This is a much more complex and interesting analytic point (which may be compared and contrasted, for example, between Trusts) than simply reporting the anxiety shown by Participant 1.*

So, when analysing focus group data, it must be emphasised that the important subjects are not necessarily the ones that get talked about most frequently (Krueger and Casey, 2000). Also, often it is when concluding questions are asked, such as 'all things considered' or 'is there anything else you'd like to add?' that participants identify the most important issues explicitly. Frequently, when the tape recording is stopped people will continue and give data that are highly relevant. Similarly, it is important to give attention to the personal context that participants use in giving their responses to the topics (Merton et al., 1990; Green and Hart, 1999).

Sim (1998) identifies three issues concerning the use of focus group data:

1. The data you obtain relate to a group rather than to a collection of separate individuals. If a focus group arrives at an apparent consensus, it is difficult to conclude that individual participants hold this view. Group interactions are complex and can lead to individual participants apparently agreeing with a view that they do not privately hold.
2. Similarly, it is problematic to measure strength of opinion in a group in the same way as in individual surveys. While particular views may be present or absent across different focus groups, the relative strength of opinion is difficult to compare.
3. Attempting to make generalisations based upon focus group data is misguided; for example, concluding that the opinions expressed by a particular group of nurses can be taken as representative of nurses as a profession.

One of the practical issues that can be challenging when transcribing focus group data is identifying which participant was speaking at any particular time. In the transcript in the case study above, each participant is given a separate number to identify them. When you are transcribing a focus group, you may find that you hear someone making a statement but it is unclear which participant it is. This can be significant during data analysis when you are trying to establish how important particular topics are. For example, a particular topic may be mentioned three times during a focus group. It is important to establish whether the point was made by three different people or whether it is the same person making the point three times. The simplest way to address this is to ensure that you have a second person who is taking notes while you moderate the focus group, because they can take notes about the order in which people spoke and help you identify participants when the recording is unclear.

Before we move on to consider the use of content analysis in documentary sources, have a go at the activity below.

Activity 5.1 — *Critical thinking*

Imagine that you are a student who is interested in exploring the impact on older people of moving into residential care. You are deciding who to interview and are considering interviewing a service user, a relative, a care manager, a care assistant and a residential home manager. What problems may this raise for data analysis?

There is a brief outline answer at the end of the chapter.

Chapter summary

In this chapter, we have discussed the processes involved in analysing qualitative data as well as a quantitative technique for analysing documents. Thematic analysis has been presented as a clear and systematic model for analysing qualitative data using a six-stage approach. Clarity and consistency are required in data analysis. These ideas can help inform your thinking when considering proposal writing and reading research reports that have used these techniques.

Activity answer

Activity 5.1: Critical thinking (page 95)

This activity looks at problems in data analysis commentary.

Although you would gain a considerable breadth of views, it would be very difficult to develop an interview schedule and to analyse the interview data. This is because all of the participants have very different roles so it would be quite challenging to devise questions that would be relevant to all participants. It would be equally challenging to analyse participants' answers because there may be few similarities between the accounts. It could be similar to trying to write an essay in which you compare the colour red, the number seven and the country Belgium (Thurlow-Brown, 1988). It also raises ethical issues because it is very difficult to anonymise participants' comments if you have chosen people from different agencies. For example, if you interview one person from a particular agency, you may present your findings as 'the participant from the voluntary agency stated that . . .'. Since there is only one participant from a voluntary agency, it is often easy for readers who are familiar with the agencies to be able to identify the staff member who is being referred to. It is more realistic to choose a smaller number of perspectives, such as service users and carers or care managers and residential staff, in order to ensure that your data can be analysed and reported in a straightforward way.

Further reading

Braun, V and Clarke, V (2006) Using thematic analysis in psychology. *Qualitative Research in Psychology*, 3: 77–101.
A comprehensive and well-written article that covers the theoretical and pragmatic issues around thematic analysis and presents a clear and detailed account of the process.

Braun, V and Clarke, V (2013) *Successful Qualitative Research: A Practical Guide for Beginners*, London: Sage.
A good qualitative research textbook with excellent coverage of data analysis.

Bryman, A (2012) *Social Research Methods*, 3rd edition. Oxford: Oxford University Press.
Good discussion of qualitative analysis and an excellent all-round research textbook.

Miles, MB and Huberman, AM (1994) *Qualitative Data Analysis: An Expanded Sourcebook*, 2nd edition. London: Sage.
Classic and highly influential textbook that provides a good background to qualitative data analysis.

Useful websites

http://onlineqda.hud.ac.uk
Online QDA provides a set of learning materials for those beginning to use Computer Assisted Qualitative Data Analysis (CAQDAS) packages as well as manual forms of data analysis. It is based at Huddersfield University and is closely connect to the CAQDAS Networking Project.

http://caqdas.soc.surrey.ac.uk
The CAQDAS Networking Project provides practical support, training and information in the use of a range of software programs designed to assist with qualitative data analysis. It is based at Surrey University and works closely with Online QDA (see above).

Chapter 6
Using and critiquing research methods: surveys and experimental designs

Chapter aims

After reading this chapter, you should be able to:

- describe the features of surveys;
- describe the features of experimental designs;
- understand the key issues of validity and reliability in surveys and in experimental designs;
- be aware of the ethical issues around experimental research.

Introduction

In this chapter we will look at common quantitative study designs: we will first consider features of questionnaire surveys, and then move on to experimental and quasi-experimental designs, including randomised controlled trials (RCTs) and related basic study designs. Issues of validity and reliability will be considered, as will sample size and power calculation. We will start from the perspective of choosing potential strategies when planning a proposal and will make reference to aspects that are important when critiquing research findings.

Survey designs

Questionnaires are a popular and widely used research method, which is at least partly because we are familiar with their use in everyday life and with the underlying principle of considering information that has been obtained from a sample of people to be representative of a much larger group of people.

Questionnaires originate from the survey tradition, which has a long history in the social sciences. The terms 'questionnaire' and 'survey' are often used interchangeably. *Surveys* are used to study large groups or populations, usually using a standardised, quantitative approach to identify beliefs, attitudes, behaviour and other characteristics. Questionnaires form a key research method for collecting survey data, but surveys can use a range of methods, such as highly structured, face-to-face or telephone interviews. Consequently, surveys are an overall research design, whereas questionnaires are one of the research methods used within surveys.

Surveys can be cross-sectional or longitudinal. A cross-sectional survey would be administered at one point in time only to assess views or attributes of a sample. Longitudinal surveys would be administered once and then again at a later date, maybe several times, to assess how the sample's views were changing or developing.

The long tradition of survey research has led to a considerable amount of rules and guidance about constructing and administering questionnaires. This chapter aims to address the key issues in questionnaire research to enable you to understand them and consider whether they might be the most appropriate method for answering your research questions and so be useful in your proposals.

We will discuss when it is appropriate to use questionnaires compared to other research methods. A five-stage model of developing questionnaire research will be presented, from deciding on a research question and design through to analysing the data. In this process, ethical issues and sampling strategies will be explored and the strengths and limitations of questionnaires will be discussed. A case study, activities and practical tips will be provided to illustrate issues in the management of a questionnaire research project.

When is it appropriate to use questionnaires?

Questionnaires are most appropriate when straightforward quantitative information is required, from a large number of people, on a relatively well-understood topic. For a topic requiring more exploratory research using data that are complex and uncertain from a smaller number of people, qualitative research methods such as interviews and focus groups may be more appropriate.

Consider the following case study.

Case study: Choosing a design

Varsha is a final-year student who is interested in her fellow nurses' experiences of their pre-registration education. She is considering two research questions:

1. *Do nursing students feel that their programme is preparing them for professional practice?*
2. *How do nursing students use theory to respond to complex practice situations?*

Activity 6.1 _Decision making_

Put yourself in Varsha's position. Which question do you think would be more appropriate for using questionnaires? Write a rationale for your answer.

There is a brief outline answer at the end of the chapter.

When planning to use a questionnaire, one of the most common mistakes is to include a significant number of open-ended, qualitative questions. This is problematic for two reasons. First, participants are unlikely to fill out the questionnaire completely because they do not want to keep writing long passages, so some questions will be ignored and participants may give up part way through. Second, it can be difficult to understand the answers they give as participants may respond to a question in very different ways and there is no opportunity to clarify responses with participants, unlike other methods such as interviews and focus groups. This may result in significant amounts of missing or confusing data. Consequently, it is best to keep the number of open-ended questions to an absolute minimum (Bryman, 2012).

Research summary

The most famous example of using open-ended, qualitative questions inappropriately comes from Karl Marx, whose workers' survey (*enquête ouvrière*) was a questionnaire sent out to 25,000 French socialists and others. It had 101 questions, finishing with the following question:

> *What is the general, physical, intellectual and moral condition of men and women employed in your trade?*
> (Bottomore and Rubel, 1963, page 218)

Unsurprisingly, there is no record of any questionnaires being returned!

The five stages of completing a questionnaire survey

The process of completing a questionnaire survey consists of five stages:

1. deciding a research question and design;
2. developing a questionnaire, including ethical issues;
3. sampling;
4. data collection;
5. data analysis.

Stage 1: Deciding a research question and design

This stage involves deciding a research question and if there is a specific hypothesis to be tested. A *hypothesis* is *a statement about the relationship between two or more variables and predicts an expected outcome* (Hek and Moule, 2006, page 58). It is a hunch coming from a reading of the literature, a theory or observations and experience and it must be capable of being tested (Nardi, 2006).

As questionnaires are most often and most effectively used in quantitative research, variables should be identified that are most relevant to the research question. *Variables* are attributes that can take on different values with different cases and could include your participants' attitudes, beliefs, behaviour, knowledge or some other characteristic. We shall follow through this process with Varsha as she develops her research project.

Case study: Using questionnaires

Varsha is interested in using questionnaires to study her fellow students' attitudes towards their professional training. She wants to know whether nursing students believe that their educational programme is preparing them for the realities of working as qualified professionals. She is interested in whether participants' responses differ according to year of study, age, gender and amount of pre-qualifying experience.

In the case study, Varsha may have a hypothesis that older students will report higher levels of confidence in their ability to practise. How might she test this? If she demonstrates that her hypothesis can be supported, will it show that older students are more prepared to practise after their training?

If she includes questions about students' age and scaling questions asking students how confident they feel in their nursing practice, she will be able to test this hypothesis. With regard to the second question, remember that Varsha's project is a survey of the attitudes of student nurses rather than an observation of their practice. Consequently, proving her hypothesis means that older students are more likely to report feeling confident about being prepared to practise. The question of whether they are actually more prepared for practice is a different question, but this is not the focus of her study.

Operationalisation, validity and reliability

The process of deciding which indicators to use when measuring variables is called *operationalisation*; that is, how to convert an abstract concept into a quantifiable measure. For example, Varsha wants to measure how confident student nurses are about their practice and has chosen to use a rating scale completed by students because it is specific and measurable. She wants to see the relationship between this and the students' year of study, age and gender.

Two key concepts when choosing the indicators to be measured are validity and reliability. *Validity* refers to whether what we are measuring is what we think we are measuring. *Reliability* refers to how consistent or stable a particular measure is. To use an example, imagine that Varsha wanted to measure how confident student nurses are and decided that the best way to do this is by measuring their physical height. Since height is not a measurement of confidence, this would not be a valid measure because she would not be measuring what she thinks she is measuring. However, assuming she used an ordinary tape measure, it could be a reliable measurement in the sense that she would measure students repeatedly and receive the same results. But if she used a tape measure made out of elastic, it would be neither valid nor reliable because she would receive different results at different times!

It is a difficult thing to develop questionnaires that are valid and reliable from scratch and as a general rule for project planning and proposal writing it is better to use instruments that are pre-existing and have been tested by researchers and found to be valid and reliable using the measures outlined in Table 6.1. There are numerous ratings scales, covering many aspects of human experience, and a quick search of the internet or of relevant academic journals in your field should find suitable ones. It may be that your programme requires you to design a questionnaire, so check before you use existing instruments. Also, it may be appropriate to develop a questionnaire as part of a project you are planning if there isn't one already in existence, and some of the issues are mentioned below. Issues of validity and reliability are addressed in Table 6.1.

Reliability		
Type	**Explanation**	**Means**
Stability	Shows that a measure is unchanging over time	Administering the test to a group once, then again later, to see if the scores are the same. Known as the test–retest method; there should be a high degree of statistical correlation between the scores
Internal reliability	Tests whether the measures are coherent and meaningful in large items scales where there are large numbers of items or questions	The split-half method: splits the scale in half, then measures whether responses are similar in magnitude in each half, so do those who score highly in one half do so in the other? This generates a correlation coefficient. Chronbach's alpha calculates the average of all possible correlation coefficients. An acceptable value is 0.8 (range 0–1)
Interobserver consistency or interrater reliability	Most simply understood as the extent to which two or more people would score (or rate) things	Most easily established by making sure there is consistency between observers, possibly by training
Validity		
Type	**Explanation**	**Means**
Face validity	Achieved by demonstrating that questions or items appear to measure the concept in question	Asking expert opinion to judge the items
Content validity	Measures the extent to which items in a rating scale measure all the key aspects of the concept in question	Similar to face validity but more powerful as face validity is based on expert opinion rather than more rigorous measurement

(Continued)

(Continued)

Concurrent validity	Comparing a criterion on which attitudes are known to differ	Measure whether attitudes do indeed differ. For example, if a new measure of job satisfaction found that attitudes to absenteeism were the same amongst those who liked and disliked their jobs, doubt may be cast on the items as it is likely that those who like their jobs regard absenteeism differently from those who don't
Predictive validity	Comparing a criterion on which attitudes are believed will differ in the future	How well does the new measure predict future absenteeism?
Construct validity	Seeks to establish how items in a new scale compare with what has been written from a theoretical point of view: the literature might suggest a relationship between variables, but does the new measure actually show this?	Correlations would be used as statistical tests to show how far the new measures fitted with existing ideas: if we believe that happy workers are absent less, does our measure show this?
Convergent validity	How well do different sources of data on an issue agree or disagree?	Using measures of attitudes collected through different means

Table 6.1: Establishing reliability and validity in questionnaires, instruments and rating scales (adapted from Bryman, 2012)

These factors will need to be acknowledged and discussion presented about how you will establish one or more of the criteria for reliability and validity in any questionnaire you plan as part of your proposal. It is not simply enough to design your own, on your own, without reference to these issues. If you still plan to use one because it meets the needs of your research question, read on for further practical issues in questionnaire design.

Stage 2: Developing a questionnaire for an undergraduate project or dissertation

The process of developing a questionnaire requires consideration of the layout, the questions to be asked and the order in which they appear on the questionnaire. It is generally recognised that having an attractive layout is important to ensure a good response rate. A poorly designed and visually unappealing questionnaire is more likely to be consigned to the waste paper bin or deleted from the e-mail inbox, so it is worthwhile investing time in getting it right.

'How long should a questionnaire be?' is a common student question. The golden rule is that questionnaires should *include as many questions as necessary and as few as possible* (Sarantakos, 2005, page 242).

Activity 6.2   *Reflection*

Think about your own experiences of filling out questionnaires. What were the best and worst parts? How long were you prepared to spend on completing a questionnaire?

When thinking about issues of questionnaire length and design, it can be useful to think about what it would be like to be the participant completing it. Most participants are prepared to spend between 5 and 15 minutes to complete a questionnaire. If a questionnaire requires considerably more time, the response rate is lower and there will be more partially completed questionnaires.

As this is a reflective exercise, there is no outline answer at the end of the chapter.

Choosing questions

When thinking of questions to be included in a questionnaire, researchers may begin by generating a range of possible questions, either alone or preferably with other people who have an interest in your research topic but who are not going to be participants. Questions generated will be reviewed and those that are not relevant discarded.

Next, they will be divided into two groups: 'need to know' and 'nice to know' (Krueger and Casey, 2000). 'Need to know' questions are vital to answering the research question whereas 'nice to know' questions are ones that are simply interesting. If all the 'nice to know' questions are included, a questionnaire will be so long that it is unlikely that many participants will ever reach the end and data will not be relevant to the research question.

Questions are traditionally divided into closed and open-ended questions. Closed questions provide participants with a fixed number of responses, while open-ended questions allow participants to respond in their own words. Closed questions with a fixed number of responses produce quantitative data that are easy to analyse.

Many of the principles of developing questions are similar to those suggested for interviews and focus groups. Ensure that questions are clear and unambiguous, without confusion and vagueness. Questions containing two elements should be avoided, such as 'did you enjoy your lectures and your practice placement?' Participants may have different responses to different parts of the question, so are likely to respond to one part only. Participants provide more reliable responses to questions that relate to their own direct experience rather than more general questions that encourage speculation and generalisations. Questions that require memory recall should be realistic.

Questions should not be repetitive. It is quite common for the initial drafts of questionnaires to ask the same question in different forms, which is confusing to participants. Language that is particularly emotional or value-laden should be avoided, as should leading questions (i.e. questions that suggest a particular response). Piloting draft questionnaires is very useful. Ensure that questions are clear and free from jargon and abbreviations (e.g. 'how did your course prepare you to meet the new NMC standards?'). These are likely to antagonise participants.

Asking 'why' questions is generally discouraged in questionnaire research. 'Why' questions suggest to participants that they should provide a rational response to what might be a decision based upon impulse, habit, tradition or other non-rational processes (Krueger and Casey, 2000). If so, participants are likely to provide an intellectual rationalisation that bears little relation to the real process.

Avoid negative questions, particularly double negatives. Participants often accidently read negative questions as positive questions and answer them accordingly. Double negatives are simply confusing.

A final issue is whether you should offer a 'don't know' option. Bryman (2012) argues that this is problematic, particularly when you are asking a question about attitudes. Although there is a possibility that participants will choose it as an easy option, leaving it out would force participants either to select an attitude they do not hold or not answer the question at all.

Deciding question order

Different sections of the questionnaire should flow like a conversation, following a logical order, and move from the familiar to the least familiar to enable participants to begin with what they know best. More objective questions should come first and move to more subjective questions as participants become more comfortable. Sensitive questions should be left to later in the questionnaire, but not at the end. As participants can become tired, have fairly straightforward questions at the end, such as participants' age, gender and ethnicity.

One technique that can aid the development of rating scales is factor analysis. This is a complex technique and in writing a proposal you would not be expected to get to grips with it, but it is common to see studies in academic journals using factor analysis. It is used to refine rating scales where there are many items (questions) by a procedure which indicates where these items tend to group together in clusters (factors) of similar ideas. This could indicate that the items in the scale have an inherent structure. So, for example, in a draft scale with 100 questions these might fall into four factors each containing 15 items (60 items in total). The remaining 40 may be barely relevant and could be discarded. Thus a potentially 100-item-long questionnaire or rating scale would be reduced to a smaller 60. The four factors would be given names relating to their content, which would add structure and also indicate key theoretical aspects of the concepts being studied (Bryman, 2012).

Choosing the format for responses

You can choose a number of different formats for how you want participants to respond (Sarantakos, 2005; Sharp, 2009). Whichever response format is used, it is essential to give clear instructions to participants about how questions should be answered:

- Exact responses: these require a specific answer (e.g. the number of pre-qualifying years of social work experience).
- Category responses: these require participants to select one response from a list of categories (e.g. pre-qualifying experience expressed as 0–2 years, 3–4 years).
- Dichotomous responses: these are usually in the form of yes/no answers, but could be other dichotomous responses (e.g. male/female).
- Likert scale questions: these usually require participants to select a response along a sliding scale of agreement. The most common format for a Likert scale is to have two extreme positions divided by a five-point scale, though a seven-point scale can be used to distinguish subtle gradations.
- Semantic differential scale: two opposite adjectives are placed on a numerical scale and participants choose which number best represents their view.
- Graphic scales: graphic representations, such as faces or ladders, are used to represent participants' attitudes. These are commonly used in learning disability research and can be particularly helpful with children. Visual analogue scales (VASs) are also popular in, for example, pain assessment. Patients may be asked to rate their pain from 0 to 100, with 100 being the most severe ever. After the administration of analgesia, if the patient were asked to re-rate the pain, the effectiveness of the analgesia could be assessed.
- Constant-sum scales and pie charts: participants are asked to score two or more alternatives so that the scores add up to a fixed amount or are presented with a blank pie chart and asked to divide it up to represent the relative importance of particular elements.

A key factor in determining what format you wish to use is how you are going to analyse the data afterwards. Consequently, it is worthwhile reading this section alongside Chapter 7, which describes some of the statistical tests that you can use with your data and some of the limitations of particular types of data. If data analysis is not planned, there is a danger that the data will be collected in a form that does not allow the use of statistical procedures required.

Let us look at Varsha's questionnaire as an example (Figure 6.1).

Varsha's questionnaire uses a wider range of questions than you would normally find, but this is to illustrate the different formats that are available. It is important to have some variety in the types of questions that you ask rather than simply having one type (e.g. yes/no answers).

This questionnaire will ask you about your nursing course.

About your course

1. **Which year of the nursing degree are you currently in?**

First	Second	Third
☐	☐	☐
1	*2*	*3*

2. **Your confidence about specific skills and areas of knowledge**
   Please tick ✓ the box that is closest to your opinion.

I feel confident about ...	Strongly agree	Agree	Neither agree nor disagree	Disagree	Strongly disagree
My listening and communication skills	☐	☐	☐	☐	☐
My ability to complete an assessment competently	☐	☐	☐	☐	☐
My clinical skills	☐	☐	☐	☐	☐
My ability to apply nursing theories in practice	☐	☐	☐	☐	☐
My knowledge of the specialist area in which I'm placed	☐	☐	☐	☐	☐
Code	*5*	*4*	*3*	*2*	*1*

3. **Overall, how would you rate how confident you feel about your ability to practise nursing competently?**
   Please put a number between 1 and 10 in the box (1 = very unconfident, 10 = very confident)

   Comment

4. Overall, to what extent do you agree or disagree that your nursing degree is preparing you for professional practice?
Please tick ✓ one box only

	Strongly agree	Agree	Neither agree nor disagree	Disagree	Strongly disagree
	☐	☐	☐	☐	☐
Code	*5*	*4*	*3*	*2*	*1*

5. How important have the following parts of your training been to your professional development?

You have 100 positive points to divide between the following elements of your course to show how important they are to your professional development. How would you allocate them? *Insert a score against each element, which should add up to 100.*

Lectures/seminars	+
Private study	+
Placement	___
Total	=100

6. Which area do you wish to work in once you have qualified?
Please describe the area in less than 10 words

```
┌─────────────────────────────────────┐
│                                      │
│                                      │
│                                      │
└─────────────────────────────────────┘
```

About you

This information is collected to see whether there are differences between the views of different people. All information will be kept confidential.

7. Are you female or male?
Please tick ✓ one box only

Female	Male
☐	☐
1	*2*

8. What was your age at your last birthday?
Please write in box

9. How many years of nursing experience did you have when you started your degree?
Please write in box

Figure 6.1: Excerpt from Varsha's questionnaire

Ethical issues

There are ethical issues to be addressed when using questionnaires, though questionnaires are generally regarded as having lower ethical risks than more intrusive research methods. Unlike interviews and focus groups, questionnaires offer the possibility of anonymity because the researcher may not know the identity of participants, which is a higher level of protection than confidentiality. This makes questionnaires useful for researching sensitive topics because participants are more likely to disclose sensitive material if they can remain anonymous. Promising anonymity is problematic if questionnaires are returned via e-mail as the researcher will usually be able to identify participants, but you will always be able to offer confidentiality.

It is common practice for questionnaires not to require written consent forms, since consent can be implied by participants completing and returning the questionnaire. However, participants do require information about the research, which is normally contained in information sheets or covering letters. You may have to go through the NHS Research Ethics Service, local NHS Trust research governance processes and a university ethics committee for approval prior to commencing the research.

Stage 3: Sampling

The next stage is deciding how you are going to select the sample. *Sampling* refers to the process of selecting the participants that will be involved in the study. The sample of participants is chosen from the total possible group of people, known as the *population*.

The two main types of sampling are probability and non-probability sampling.

Probability or *random sampling* uses mathematical techniques based upon probability theory to select research participants who are representative of the overall population. It is the most common sampling approach used in questionnaire research and random sampling increases the likelihood that the results will be generalisable to a wider population. Non-probability sampling is a weaker form of sampling, but is still used in many studies for convenience (hence convenience sampling).

Samples can be divided up (or stratified) in certain ways, such as age, gender and ethnicity, although this may not be necessary, particularly if the resultant sample size is relatively small. For example, having one or two people from a specific ethnic group is too small a sample size to be able to make any worthwhile generalisations. In research, it is always wise to be realistic about what can be claimed based upon evidence and it is better to understate rather than overstate a case.

Choosing the sample is important, as it will influence the data received. A famous example is the *Chicago Daily Tribune* erroneously announcing that Republican Thomas Dewey had won the US presidential election in 1948, rather than Democrat Harry Truman. This occurred because the newspaper had seen polls that predicted a Dewey victory, but the poll had been conducted using a biased sample. The polls were conducted using fixed quotas from rural and urban populations that had not been updated to reflect the recent move from rural areas into cities. Consequently, they underrepresented urban voters who were more likely to vote for Democrat Truman (Andersen and Taylor, 2005, page 42).

Bryman (2012) identifies four main types of probability sampling: *simple random sampling, systematic sampling, stratified random sampling* and *multi-stage cluster sampling.*

Simple random sampling

This is the most basic form of random sampling, in which cases are selected randomly using random number tables or an online random generator (such as www.randomizer.org). Each unit of the population has an equal chance of being included in the sample and this method eliminates human bias. However, it is only possible if you have a list of all people in your population (i.e. a sampling frame).

Systematic sampling

This is a variation of the simple random sample, in which cases are selected in a systematic way (e.g. choosing every tenth case). It is important to ensure the sampling frame (list of potential participants) is not structured in a way that would make it non-random and, if so, to randomise the order of the list.

Stratified random sampling

If there are particular factors to be concentrated upon, the sample can be made to ensure sufficient representation. In the case study, Varsha may be interested in whether gender makes a difference in students' attitudes about their professional programmes. She could establish the overall gender proportions in the nursing student group and choose a proportionate sample for each gender. Having established the overall target number of participants for each gender, she would then choose specific participants using simple random sampling or systematic sampling.

Multi-stage cluster sampling

When a sample is geographically spread, cluster sampling enables the grouping together of potential participants. Imagine that Varsha wanted to research nursing students across the UK. It would be unrealistic to sample randomly every student, as that would need students from every university. Instead, cluster sampling would enable her to choose a smaller number of universities through random sampling. She may wish to group the universities further (e.g. choosing regions) and randomly select them within specific regions (Bryman, 2012).

Stage 4: Data collection

Having developed a questionnaire, it is important to pilot it because, unlike interviews or focus groups, there is no opportunity to explain ambiguous or unclear questions. Questions that make sense to the authors may not make sense to participants, who may consistently misread questions, so such questions need to be reworded.

One aim is to maximise your response rate. Having developed a clear and attractive questionnaire, the response rate can be improved by using follow-up letters with additional copies of the questionnaire. This can be fruitful, but should not delay a project too much. A general rule of thumb is that about three-quarters of completed questionnaires should be returned in the first three weeks. The final quarter may respond to a reminder letter, but there will come a point when the project must proceed to the next stage. Distributing questionnaires by e-mail makes the whole process of administering them and sending reminders much easier and cheaper.

Stage 5: Analysing your data and presenting your findings

The analysis of your data using descriptive statistics will be discussed in detail in Chapter 7. It would be worthwhile reading this now to understand how data collection progresses to analysis.

Strengths and limitations of questionnaires

Questionnaires have a number of strengths and weaknesses (Sarantakos, 2005; Bryman, 2012).

Their strengths are as follows:

- Questionnaires are relatively inexpensive and quick to administer.
- Participants can respond when it is convenient for them and there is a greater assurance of anonymity.
- There are fewer opportunities for errors or bias caused by the presence of the interviewer. For example, participants may give answers that are sociably acceptable but not accurate (social desirability bias).
- The questions are asked in a stable and consistent manner, with no interviewer variability. They allow greater coverage because participants can be approached more easily and there are no problems around 'non-contacts', where participants are not available at the time (Sarantakos, 2005).

Their weaknesses are as follows:

- Questionnaires do not allow opportunities for probing and clarifying responses with participants, or for collecting additional information (e.g. observation) while the questionnaire is being completed.
- The researcher does not have an opportunity to motivate the participant to complete all of the questions or ensure the questions are answered in the correct order, if relevant.
- There are limitations as to how long participants are willing to spend on completing a questionnaire.
- Only a very limited number of open questions can be asked, because participants do not want to write large amounts.
- They are less appropriate for people with literacy difficulties or for whom English is not a first language.
- The identity of the participant is not known, so the researcher cannot be sure the right person has completed the questionnaire.
- Non-response or a low response rate hinders the analysis and interpretation of results.

Experimental designs

An experimental approach involves setting up a research study in which the outcome is not known (Donnan, 2000). The intention is to compare the effects of some new treatment or procedure administered to one group of patients with those in another group receiving either 'normal care' or a placebo (and so do not experience anything novel). The study is designed to test researchers' hypotheses, or research questions, about the effectiveness of the new treatment. The RCT is often described as the gold standard in this type of research; this approach is able to indicate as closely as possible whether or not hypotheses are correct when conducted in a rigorous fashion (although the accuracy of this term is disputed by, for example, Cartwright (2007)). If there was no control or comparison group, it is possible that participants might gain benefit just because something new is being done to them; the mind can produce all kinds of physical and psychological responses to treatments and placebos. The Hawthorne effect occurs when an effect noted in a research study could occur because participants know they are involved in the study (Hek and Moule, 2006). Thus a control group is needed to assess whether the new treatment works over and above any possible Hawthorne effect.

Essential features of a randomised controlled trial

For a study to be a true experiment, the following features apply (Donnan, 2000; Tilling et al., 2005; Williamson et al., 2010b).

Comparison and control groups

These are required to test a hypothesis: variables will be manipulated and outcomes assessed between the experimental and control group(s). In this way extraneous variables are controlled out (external influences are removed so that researchers can be sure that the effects noted are due to the actions of the intervention and not some other factors) and internal validity is high.

Sampling

As it is not possible to include all potentially eligible subjects of a population, samples must be taken and these should theoretically be random samples. However, practical considerations mean that researchers often use convenience samples. Other sampling methods include cluster sampling, where groups of sites such as GP practices or hospitals would be included, and stratified random sampling, where sampling takes place to reflect some characteristic in a population such as age or sex.

Sample size and power calculations

Researchers should plan the number of participants to be recruited based on up-front calculations rather than guesswork. In a proposal you would need to demonstrate that you were aware of the importance of having the correct sample size and write about how this could be demonstrated. Having too many participants in the study exposes them to unnecessary risk; having too few runs the risk of missing statistically significant findings (type II errors). In planning a proposal as part of an undergraduate piece of work you would be unlikely to be expected to do sample size estimation and power calculations but would be expected to write coherently about what they mean and why they are important. As the Consolidated Standards of Reporting Trials (CONSORT) statement puts it:

> *The sample size for a trial needs to be planned carefully, with a balance between medical and statistical considerations. Ideally, a study should be large enough to have a high probability (power) of detecting as statistically significant a clinically important difference of a given size if such a difference exists. The size of effect deemed important is inversely related to the sample size necessary to detect it; that is, large samples are necessary to detect small differences.*
> (Moher et al., 2010, page 8)

What this means is that researchers, in advance, should work out the numbers they require and the effect size that these numbers will be able to detect. This will typically be expressed in a short paragraph saying they calculated that (say) 100 participants were required in each group to detect a clinically significant effect with a power of, for example, 0.8 at an α level of 0.05 (α corresponds to the p value and indicates the acceptable risk of chance findings or type I errors, set by convention at 0.05 or 5% – more on this in Chapter 7); 0.8 power (or 80%) indicates the power that the study has to determine the effect size. The desired level of chance in the clinical results will be dependent on what is under study, and researchers will determine what a large or small effect size is relative to their study and existing literature. To gain the precision to detect relatively small changes, relatively large samples will be required.

Eligibility of subject

Clear protocols should indicate inclusion and exclusion criteria (such as age and sex) for participants, to ensure that those enrolled in the study are appropriate and the sample is relatively homogeneous.

Fully informed consent

One key aspect of the practicalities of undertaking an RCT is the extent to which informed consent can be gained; without informed consent the study would be unethical. So, even though there may be a risk of harm to the patients in some new treatment, or less beneficial outcomes if they are in the placebo group, if this is explained and patients still consent then these risks are acceptable.

Randomisation

Once the sample has been chosen, is it practically and/or ethically possible to randomise participants between groups? Researchers randomly split participants between one or more study groups to avoid accidental or intentional biases in the different study groups. The groups will then be compared and their characteristics assessed to make sure there are no biases in the group allocations. For example, if we were testing a new treatment for high blood pressure (hypertension) we would want to make sure that the mean (average) blood pressure at the start of the study in each group was similar: if our intervention group had a much lower mean blood pressure before starting the new treatment compared to the group continuing to take their existing treatment, then this would be reflected in the study findings. An element of accidental bias would have been introduced at the sampling stage and the findings would show that those in the treatment group had a lower blood pressure than the others. Similarly, randomisation of patients into different groups prevents the researchers from introducing intentional biases which may show their study in a more favourable light if they hand-picked the 'best' participants. Methods of randomisation include simple randomisation, where random numbers are generated to allocate participants between groups; block randomisation, where participants are allocated a block and these are then split between treatment and control, to ensure that numbers allocated to each group are similar; and stratified randomisation, to ensure that characteristics such as age and sex are allocated evenly between groups.

Blinding of treatment

It should be impossible for patients, staff and researchers to know who is receiving the new treatment and who is not. This is known as double-blinding and is to avoid intentional and unintentional biases being introduced to findings if participants were treated differently because of the group they were in, or responded differently to treatment because of their own perceptions of how they were being treated. If double-blinding is not possible, a study may go ahead but it must be acknowledged that these potential biases may exist and overestimate the effects of treatment.

Analysis of differences between research or control groups

Using appropriate statistical tests and software (a common package is SPSS, the Statistical Package for the Social Sciences), statistical significance is indicated by the use of p values and/or confidence intervals (CIs) and indicates the generalisabilty of the study findings by assessing how far the results from the study sample might relate to the larger population. This will be discussed more fully in Chapter 7 on data analysis.

Limitations of RCTs

Although they may be the gold standard, even RCTs have their weaknesses and some of these are outlined below (Donnan, 2000; Tilling et al., 2005; Williamson et al., 2010b):

- Non-compliance: if participants do not routinely comply with the new treatment regime it is likely that the effects will be understated.
- Drop-out rates: if patients do not complete the study then their data will be lost and outcomes will not be fully assessed. This may be because of side-effects of the new treatment, voluntary withdrawal or death. This can be avoided by using intention-to-treat analysis, which means that all patients who began the study are included, and gives a pragmatic estimate of the effects of treatment policy rather than the actual outcomes of the study. (For a fuller explanation of this concept, see Hollis and Campbell, 1999.)
- Statistical significance may be established, but are the results clinically important and can they be applied in the real world (are they clinically effective)? It is not a flaw if a study

reports no statistically significant differences between active and control groups in an RCT, provided the study has been correctly conducted and is adequately powered. It may be as clinically useful to know that a new treatment or procedure does not work as it is to know that it does.

- RCTs tell us nothing on their own about the patient's experience, and sometimes 'nested qualitative studies' may be included in RCTs to gain this type of information.

There are many different types of experimental designs, and these are noted in Table 6.2. A trial would be called a quasi-experimental design if some feature such as randomisation or group concealment (double-blinding) was not possible. A quasi-experiment would also be possible if there were naturally occurring groups, such as patients already receiving some treatment. In this case, researchers would not be manipulating variables, but would be choosing the timing and extent of measurement that takes place (Punch, 2005). As a result, these would be less robust designs as if, for example, patients and staff could easily identify which group they were in (double-blinding was absent) they might be able consciously or unconsciously to influence outcomes.

Design	Key features	Advantages	Disadvantages
Randomised controlled trial	Participants randomly allocated to intervention or control arm (can be placebo or 'usual treatment')	Groups balanced in everything except treatment received. If randomisation concealed, can prevent selection bias and undue potential influence from researchers	Time and effort required to make the study robust and to implement it effectively
Cluster randomised controlled trial	Groups of participants (e.g. GP practices or clusters of hospital trusts in different areas) randomised to intervention or control	Logistically easier and more suitable for some interventions (e.g. community education programmes)	Need larger sample size than individually randomised trials
Controlled trial	Participants non-randomly assigned to intervention or control arm	Easier to carry out than a randomised trial, as no need to prepare and conceal randomised allocation schedule	Allocation schedule cannot be concealed, so selection bias may occur

Before/after comparison	Data collected before and after an intervention on a group of participants, and a paired comparison made	Reduces variability by using paired data	Changes other than the experimental intervention may occur over the time period
Randomised crossover trial	As above, but each participant receives control and intervention treatment in random order. Paired comparison made	Reduces variability by using paired data	Unsuitable for interventions with long-term effects, or conditions that change over time
Historical	Data collected after an intervention and compared to data collected on some other group which did not experience the intervention. Unpaired comparison made	Requires minimal data	There may be differences between the intervention arm and the historical controls other than the experimental intervention

Table 6.2: Randomised and non-randomised experimental designs (adapted from Tilling et al., 2005)

Planning for analysis

As well as discussion of the key features above, a project plan for an RCT would need to contain specific information on how the numerical data were to be analysed, including what variables were to be assessed and what statistical tests would be used to test for differences between the intervention and the control group. Issues of sampling and data analysis contribute to the external validity of experimental designs and the generalisabilty of findings from the sample to the wider population. In a large measure this is their 'point': to show whether or not findings in the sample are likely to apply to all others with the condition.

A proposal should include a diagram showing the key stages, and with the stages clearly outlined. This allows readers to assess its replicability (Bryman, 2012). The CONSORT statement (Moher et al., 2010; and see the CONSORT website: www.consort-statement.org/home) provides an excellent example of how the study should be mapped out, with key stages (Moher et al., 2010) presented in Figure 6.2.

Figure 6.2: CONSORT 2010 flow diagram. Reproduced from Moher et al. (2010)

In proposals, as no actual participants have been recruited, only the stages of enrolment and allocation can be completed as there will be no follow-up or analysis, as shown in the box below (adapted from Moher et al., 2010).

Enrolment and allocation for proposals

1. Numbers of eligible subjects:

   (a) excluded ($n =$)
   (b) meets/does not meet inclusion criteria ($n =$)
   (c) declined to take part ($n =$)
   (d) other reasons ($n =$)

2. Randomised between groups ($n =$)

3.   Allocation:

   (a) allocated to intervention or control groups (*n* =)
   (b) received intervention or control (*n* =)
   (c) did not receive intervention or control (reasons) (*n* =)

It is imperative that researchers writing proposals for RCTs access this CONSORT website as it is an internationally recognised consensus on planning and reporting RCTs with lots of valuable resources.

Ethical issues

In proposals, there needs to be more depth about ethical issues. We have outlined key concerns of RCTs above in terms of the need for informed consent and of exposing participants to risks associated with introducing or withholding new treatments or interventions, and these would need to be more fully discussed in a proposal. One thing to consider about potential risks in RCTs from an ethical point of view is that there must be sufficient uncertainty about whether the intervention works or not to allow the trial to go ahead. If it is certain that the intervention is better than usual care a study should not proceed (Tilling et al., 2005) as there is no scientific justification for it: we already know that the intervention works best and giving another group lesser treatment is unethical. Similarly, use of placebos can be unethical and so new interventions are usually compared with 'usual care'. For example, in a study testing some new analgesic regime postsurgery, it would be unethical to trial this against a placebo as it is already well established that effective analgesic regimes exist and to expose patients to surgery without suitable postoperative pain relief would be very unpleasant for them.

Other particular ethical concerns include the vulnerability of participants. Coercion in all forms should be avoided. The relationship between clinical staff and sick people makes them more vulnerable than healthy adults, and this must be mitigated and discussed in proposals. Written consent is essential, so a written participant information sheet (PIS) and a consent form are required, and these should be included as appendices in proposals. Ethical clearance will be required from the NHS Research Ethics Service, as will local NHS Trust governance clearance and, for students, approval from the university committee.

Activity 6.3   *Critical thinking*

From Table 6.2, decide which types of study are fully experimental and which are quasi-experimental designs.

There is a brief outline answer at the end of the chapter.

> ## Chapter summary
>
> In this chapter, we have learnt about common quantitative study designs, surveys and experimental designs, and questionnaires as a research method within the survey tradition. You have been invited to consider which types of research question are appropriate to be addressed using questionnaires. A five-stage model of developing questionnaire research has been presented, taking you from deciding your research question and design through to analysing the data you have collected. We then moved on to discuss aspects of experimental designs, particularly their strengths and weaknesses. Ethical issues and sampling strategies were explored. A case study, activities and practical tips were provided in relation to questionnaires, and for experimental designs process issues were outlined and the CONSORT website strongly recommended for further information.

Activity answers

Activity 6.1: Decision making (page 98)

The first question can be answered by quantitative data that measure participants' attitudes and beliefs and a questionnaire would be ideally suited to this. The second question is more suited to qualitative methods, such as interviews and focus groups, which can provide opportunities for participants to draw upon their experiences of using theory to respond to practice situations.

Activity 6.3: Critical thinking (page 117)

From Table 6.2, decide which types of study are fully experimental and which are quasi-experimental designs:

- Fully experimental: RCT, cluster RCT, randomised crossover trial.

  o Explanation: all these have full randomisation, with concealment of group membership.

- Quasi-experimental: controlled trial, before/after comparison, historical.

  o Explanation: these do not have randomisation, or a control group.

Further reading

Bowling, A (2009) *Research Methods in Health: Investigating Health and Health Services.* Maidenhead: Open University Press.
Bowling, A and Ebrahim, S (2005) *Handbook of Research Methods in Health: Investigation, Measurement and Analysis.* Maidenhead: Open University Press.
Both of these texts are good and informative about aspects of experimental and survey designs.

De Vaus, DA (2002) *Surveys in Social Research,* 5th edition. London: Routledge.
Fifth edition of a classic text on survey research. Readable and authoritative.

Hollis, S and Campbell, F (1999) What is meant by intention to treat analysis? Survey of published randomised controlled trials. *British Medical Journal*, 319 (7211): 670–674.

Jadad, AR and Enkin, MW (2007) *Randomized Controlled Trials: Questions, Answers and Musings.* Oxford: Blackwell Publishing.
Good chapter on ethics and controlled trials.

Nezu, AM and Nezu, M (2008) *Evidence-Based Outcome Research: A Practical Guide to Conducting Randomized Controlled Trials for Psychosocial Interventions.* Oxford: Oxford University Press.
More advanced text with emphasis on psychological usage of controlled trials.

Sapsford, R (2007) *Survey Research*, 2nd edition. London: Sage.
Useful and readable text that covers the key issues in survey research.

Torgerson, DJ and Togerson, CJ (2008) *Designing Randomised Trials in Health, Education and the Social Sciences.* Basingstoke: Palgrave Macmillan.
Detailed text but useful for those looking for a more advanced text.

Useful websites

http://news.bbc.co.uk/1/hi/england/london/4807042.stm
BBC News website with information about a drug trial at Northwick Park Hospital that went wrong.

http://surveynet.ac.uk/sqb
The Survey Question Bank is part of the Survey Resources Network, an Economic and Social Research Council (ESRC) initiative coordinated by the UK Data Archive (UKDA) at the University of Essex.

www.controlled-trials.com
Information about current controlled trials.

www.drugtrial.co.uk/what-is-a-clinical-trial/how-medical-trials-are-regulated.cfm
Parexel website about how clinical trials are regulated.

http://en.wikipedia.org
Wikipedia: normally not recommended as an academic source – definitely do not quote it in assignments – but has an excellent page on clinical trials, particularly the stages that new products go through before they get to market. Google 'clinical trials' and click on the Wikipedia source, or search for clinical trials in the Wikipedia site.

Chapter 7
Analysing quantitative data and understanding basic statistics

Chapter aims

After reading this chapter, you should be able to:

- understand the basic statistical concepts and statistical tests used in quantitative studies;
- plan quantitative data analysis;
- have some ideas about how to present and interpret your results;
- know what p values, confidence intervals, relative risk and odds ratios are.

Introduction

In this chapter we will explore approaches to quantitative data, offering some practical considerations on how to plan its analysis. We will introduce some basic concepts in statistics and statistical tests used in quantitative studies. This is at an introductory level and assumes no prior knowledge of this subject. We will not be looking at complex formulae, or deep maths and statistics, but we will be introducing you to the concepts you will see discussed in papers and which you will need to plan your own proposals. We will also look at some epidemiological measures of assessing risks of disease, and a means of assessing the clinical impact of experimental studies.

Analysing quantitative data

The focus of this section is to provide some understanding of the analytic procedures based upon descriptive and inferential statistics, which will enable you to discuss how you would go about analysing quantitative data in a research proposal.

Different levels of measurement of quantitative data

In order to be able to analyse quantitative data, it is necessary to understand that there are different levels of measurement inherent in different types of variables. Although this may initially appear slightly technical, it is necessary to understand these different types of data because they are treated differently. The different levels of measurement are as follows:

- Nominal (or categorical)-level data: data placed into named categories, such as male/female, which do not have a particular order. Although numbers may be used to code nominal data, these do not have arithmetical qualities. These are the most basic forms of data and not amenable to some forms of statistical analysis.
- Ordinal-level data: data placed into categories that have an order, a relationship with each other; for example, a Likert scale on a questionnaire in which the participant chooses from 'strongly agree', 'agree', 'neutral', 'disagree', 'strongly disagree'. We can infer the rank order but not the relative size. For example, we can infer that a participant who ticks 'strongly agree' holds the opinion more intensely than one who ticks 'agree'. However, we cannot infer whether, for example, the first participant feels twice or three times as strongly as the second, only the rank order or preference.
- Interval-level data: these are similar to ordinal data but ranked on a scale with equal intervals between categories (e.g. temperature). The scale does not have a zero point anchored in the real world; for example, the Celsius scale has a zero point that is arbitrarily set at the temperature that water freezes. Interval data enable a wider range of mathematical procedures to be used.
- Ratio-level data: like interval-level data, but the categories have a scale with a true zero point, such as age or income. This is the highest level of data and enables a full range of mathematic procedures to be used.

| Activity 7.1 | *Research and finding evidence* |

Imagine you are doing a research study into the drinking habits and satisfaction of different people in different pubs. Identify from the following those variables which are nominal, ordinal, interval and ratio:

- Drinking alcohol: yes or no?
- Number of alcoholic drinks consumed
- Satisfaction with the pub bar service ('very dissatisfied', 'dissatisfied', 'neutral', 'satisfied', 'very satisfied')
- Number of men in the pub
- Number of women in the pub
- Income of each individual
- Pounds spent that evening
- Temperature in the bar area
- Would return: yes or no?
- Eating food: yes or no?
- Satisfaction with the pub food service ('very dissatisfied', 'dissatisfied', 'neutral', 'satisfied', 'very satisfied').

Answers are given at the end of the chapter.

Types of quantitative data analysis

Data can be analysed with descriptive and/or inferential statistics. Descriptive statistics are simply that: they describe the data. In many studies it is acceptable and correct only to use simple statistics like percentages or averages (means) to show the results, and conclusions can still be drawn from them. However, the growth in processing power of modern personal computers means that they are capable of running more complex operations. It has become possible for researchers to run more easily inferential statistics, and these functions are able to draw often sophisticated comparisons between variables in data. We will begin by looking at the different types of descriptive statistics that are available to you when analysing and presenting your data, and then move on to a brief indication of the types of inferential statistics that may be considered.

Simple descriptive statistics

Frequency tables enable you to show the incidence of particular responses. Percentages enable you to show figures as a proportion of the whole and can make data easier to understand.

What is the average? Measures of central tendency

Measures of central tendency report a typical or average value. The three main measures of central tendency are the mean, the median and the mode.

The *mean* is the arithmetic average, calculated by adding up the value of all of the responses and dividing by the number of responses received. It can only be used with interval and ratio data, which have true arithmetical properties. The *median* is the middle point, when data are lined up in order. If you have an even number of data, it is halfway between the two middle values. The median can be used with any type of numerical data. The *mode* is the most common response given and can be used with all four types of data.

Since different questions produce different types of data (nominal, ordinal, ratio and interval), you need to ensure that the measure of central tendency (mean, mode and median) is appropriate for the type of data you are collecting. If we apply this to Activity 7.1 above, we can see that the questionnaire produces nominal, ordinal and ratio data, which should be treated differently.

Different types of data

Nominal data

The question on drinking alcohol produces nominal data because, although numerical codes are given (yes = 1, no = 2), the data do not have arithmetical qualities. The mean cannot be used because it would be meaningless to calculate an 'average of whether drinking alcohol or not' of 1.5.

Ordinal data

The questions using Likert scales to measure whether drinkers are satisfied or not with the bar and food service produce ordinal data. If more pub goers were satisfied with the bar service than any of the other responses, the mode could be used to analyse these data, and if the scales were coded 1 for very dissatisfied up to 5 for very satisfied, the mode would be 4. It would, however, be inappropriate to work out a mean score because these are ordinal data and therefore do not have full numerical qualities; that is, the score 2 (= dissatisfied) is not twice the size of the score 4 (= satisfied).

Ratio data

The questions about the pub goers' incomes, numbers of drinks and pounds spent produce ratio data that have full numerical qualities (e.g. someone spending £20 spends twice as much as someone spending £10). Consequently, it would be appropriate to work out the mean by dividing the total sum of the spending with the number of respondents. So, for example, if total spending was £1,000 that evening and there were 100 people in the pub, the mean would be £10. The mode and median are also appropriate measures. In this example, let's assume there is no mode because no response appears more than once, but a median could be calculated. This would be done by lining up all the responses in numerical order and seeing which is the middle figure. Here is how it would be if there were 11 responses. The figures are the spending of each person in pounds:

5, 6, 8, 10, 15, 16, 17, 19, 24, 27, 29

The median is 16 because once the responses are lined up in numerical order, 16 is the middle response. Note the mean here is also 16. Medians may be used where extremes of data are in evidence as the mean is more sensitive to extremes. For example, imagine we had received these responses:

1, 6, 8, 10, 15, 16, 17, 19, 24, 47, 59

Now, the median is still 16, but the mean has shifted to 20.18 in response to the more extreme values.

Table 7.1 summarises appropriate descriptive statistics for different levels of measurement.

	Mode	**Median**	**Mean**
Nominal	✓	✗	✗
Ordinal	✓	✓	✗
Interval	✓	✓	✓
Ratio	✓	✓	✓

Table 7.1: Appropriate descriptive statistics for different levels of measurement

What is the range? Measures of dispersion

Measures of dispersion indicate the degree of variety or spread of the data. Providing averages can be helpful for understanding the midpoint of data, but it is also important to look at the spread. The simplest way is using the range, which gives the lowest and highest points. Using the first set of data for pub spending from the box above, the mean is 16, but the range is 5–29. However, this simple range only gives the first and last points, and is unreliable concerning the variability of the data, so the interquartile range can be used (Parahoo, 2006) so that, using the median value again as a middle point (Q2, below), the data set can be analysed as quartiles (split into quarters). Using the data set from above for pounds spent, it can be analysed as quartiles like this:

$$5, 6, 8, 10, 15, 16, 17, 19, 24, 27, 29$$
$$\downarrow \qquad\qquad \downarrow \qquad\qquad \downarrow$$
$$Q1 \qquad\qquad Q2 \qquad\qquad Q3$$

The interquartile range is the distance between the first and third quartiles, 8–24 (24 – 8 = 16). The semi-interquartile range is half the difference between Q1 and Q3, and in this example would be 16/2 = 8. This is the typical distance of scores from the median, and is a more useful measure in describing the data set as it goes beyond either the median or the range (Parahoo, 2006).

The most frequently used measure for describing a data set is the *standard deviation* (SD), which shows an average of how all data points differ from the mean. In our pub spending example, if the spending of each individual was relatively similar (homogeneous), then the SD would be small, zero or close to zero. If there was a great discrepancy between the pounds spent by all the pub goers (if their spending was relatively dissimilar or heterogeneous), then the SD would be larger. The exact SD will depend on all the values collected which form the data set, and will be reported with the mean value.

Normal distribution

Normal distribution is a concept that has been demonstrated to be correct and forms part of central limit theorem. It applies to many human properties, such as intelligence quotient (IQ) measurement, height and weight, and students' test scores, where most people's scores are close to the mean value, with fewer scoring extreme values. A normal distribution curve is a 'bell-shaped' curve (Figure 7.1), and it is important because many statistical tests rely on the assumption that data collected adhere to this relationship. In a normal distribution, 68% of data will fall between 1 SD of the mean, 95% of data will fall within 2 SD of the mean, 99.7% of data will fall within 3 SD of the mean and 28% will fall between 1 and 2 SD.

Representing the results

The final part of data analysis is representing the results in an acceptable manner. In the descriptive statistics discussed above, frequency tables, simple graphs and pie charts could be used.

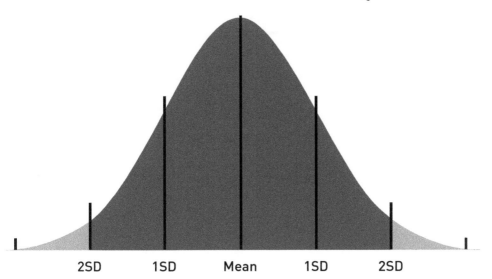

Figure 7.1: Normal distribution curve. Adapted from an original graph by Jeremy Kemp (2 September 2005)

Frequency tables (like Table 7.2) present information about the relative occurrence of different values. They are useful when information is difficult to present in graph form because the highest and lowest values are significantly different or a high level of precision is required.

Overall, how satisfied are you with the bar service at this pub?

	η	**per cent**
Very dissatisfied	6	12%
Dissatisfied	24	48%
Neutral	11	22%
Satisfied	6	12%
Very satisfied	3	6%
Total	*50*	*100%*

Table 7.2: Frequency table

Please note that the η column in Table 7.2 indicates the actual number of responses. This enables the reader to know how many responses were received and whether there were missing data. You can see from this table that this pub is not doing very well with its bar service, as 60% are either dissatisfied or very dissatisfied.

Pie charts enable you to present information about the relative proportion of different elements. They can be used when the values are added together or you have only one set of data that all have positive values. You can see from the pie chart shown in Figure 7.2 that there were 73% men in the pub, compared to 27% women.

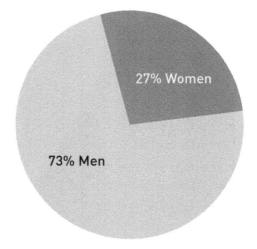

Figure 7.2: Pie chart

Bar graphs (Figure 7.3) enable you to compare data across categories. Simple bar graphs present single values and clustered bar graphs present groups of values together. In the example shown in Figure 7.3, comparing men's and women's dissatisfaction with bar service, you can see that women were more dissatisfied than men.

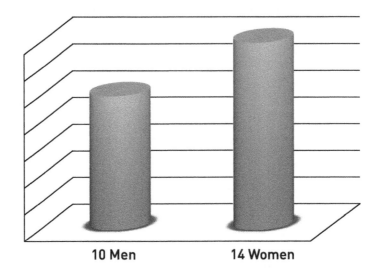

Figure 7.3: Bar graph

Inferential statistics

Descriptive statistics can be acceptable, but more interesting and important relationships can be uncovered between variables in quantitative studies using inferential statistics. It is here that hypotheses become particularly relevant, as they are tested using inferential statistics. If we have a null hypothesis, this means that there is no difference between variables, and the results are said to accept or reject that null hypothesis.

It is important to understand that inferential statistics are about estimating parameters or results in sample data. In research studies we are rarely able to gain data from an entire population, so we must sample them. Thus we may select 1,000 people to represent a population of 1,000,000, as this would be cheaper, easier and more feasible given research-funding limitations. The purpose of inferential statistical testing is therefore to give us an idea of the relationships between variables that exist in our sample, and whether these might be expected to hold true in the wider population from which the sample was drawn.

Statistical significance

Statistical significance is said to be present by convention if a test gives a value of $p < 0.05$. What this means is that there is a less than 5% chance of the results shown in the study sample being by chance, if they were repeated in the population; 5% is taken as an acceptable level of probability although others can be set. $p < 0.01$ would be a 1% chance (better); $p < 0.001$ would be a 0.01% chance (even better) of the results in the study being by accident. The p value can be between 0 and 1, and is an index of the probability of the study results being likely if the study was repeated in a population. It works inversely,

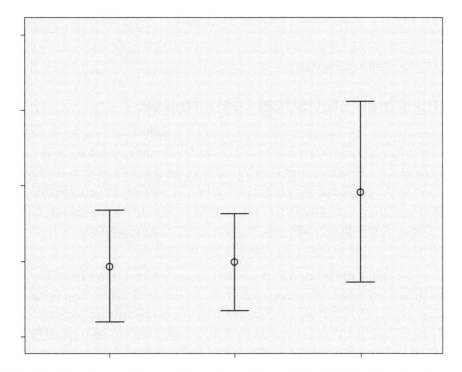

Figure 7.4: Confidence intervals containing point estimates. The right-hand one is a less precise estimate as it has a larger range. Adapted from an original graph by Sigbert (8 December 2008)

meaning that smaller is better. The *p* value does not tell us whether the study is a good one or not. Finding that there are no relationships between variables can be as interesting and relevant as finding that there are relationships. It is possible, however, that errors can be made in hypothesis testing. These can be type I and type II errors. A type I error occurs when a statistically significant relationship is found in a study where in fact it does not exist, and this might happen if the *p* value was set too high, hence the convention of $p < 0.05$. A type II error exists when no relationship is found when there is one. Either type of error can lead to the wrong conclusions being drawn about a study's results (Parahoo, 2006). (Please review the material on pages 111–112, where the importance of sample size and power have already been discussed.)

Another way of estimating statistical significance is using confidence intervals (CIs). These are ranges generated in the data from our sample between which we can be confident that the true value for the actual population will lie. By convention this is usually set at 95% (although you may see 99% CIs), meaning that our data will generate a range of values between which we can be 95% certain that the true population value lies.

In Figure 7.4, the CIs are the lines which represent a range of values. The point estimates (or summary statistics) are the dots in the middle of the lines which indicate where the values for the actual population are estimated to lie. CIs will be in the units of the study (so if we were using them in our pub analogy, the units might be pints of beer). If the summary statistic (or point estimate) falls between the CIs, then we can be 95% certain that these results represent the population and are statistically significant; if the summary statistic is outside the CIs, it is not statistically significant (Diamond and Jeffries, 2001; Peat, 2002). CIs also allow us to assess the relative precision available in the results as the wider the CI, the less precise or less accurate an estimation the results are said to be.

Deciding which statistical tests to use

In a real research project it would be necessary to obtain the help of a statistician on elements of statistical testing such as which tests to use. Local NHS Trusts usually have a research design service as part of their Research and Development Departments and statisticians should be available for consultation through them. For a proposal, you would be expected to identify your variables and the types of tests you would want to use. Obviously as you have not collected any data at this proposal stage you cannot actually run any tests. Some basic considerations in choosing which tests to use are listed in the box below.

If the data are normally distributed and the data are at interval/ratio level, then parametric statistics (which are more robust and powerful) can be used; if not, non-parametric tests are necessary (Peat, 2002). *Parametric* means that the data conform to certain assumptions, one of which is that they are normally distributed. This can be plotted in a distribution curve like the one in Figure 7.1 so that most of the data clusters around the mean, with more extreme values on the outer fringes. If data were plotted that looked exactly like Figure 7.1, they would be said to be normally distributed, but if there was a tendency for the data to cluster to the right or left of the mean, it would be said to be skewed.

Deciding on which tests to use (adapted from Peat, 2002)

1. If there is only one outcome variable

With interval/ratio variables, the following tests could be used:

- one-sample *t*-tests, paired *t*-tests (if the variable was measured at more than one point in time), analysis of variance (if measured three or more times)

With nominal-level variables:

- proportions and CIs
- McNemar's test (non-parametric, if the variables are measured more than once)

2. If there are two variables

With both interval/ratio variables:

- Pearson's *r* correlation (parametric), regression

With both nominal-level variables:

- chi-squared, odds ratios

With one nominal and one interval-level variable:

- Spearman's rho (ρ) (non-parametric correlation), logistic regression, two-sample *t*-tests, Wilcoxon test, 95% CIs

3. If there are more than two variables

- multiple regression, analysis of variance (ANOVA), factor analysis

Applications

How might these types of statistics be used in study design?

Case study: Using statistical analysis

Imagine that we are researchers working for a cosmetics company. We have developed a new type of face cream that has cost millions of pounds to get to the stage of testing on humans. As part of that process we decide to test the theory (hypothesis) that as we age we get more wrinkly.

In order to test the hypothesis that as we age we get more wrinkly, we develop a measure of wrinkles, and use it on the faces of 1,000 volunteers. Next, we run a statistical test looking at the correlations between age and wrinkliness. A correlation is a measure of association. It does not prove that one variable causes another, but indicates instead that they are associated in some way.

(continued)

continued ...

The independent variable is age, the dependent is wrinkliness (we know this to be true as there is no way it could be the other way around: wrinkliness cannot cause ageing).

As the data are found to be normally distributed and at ratio level, we use Pearson's r correlation. We enter the data into the computer program SPSS, and test age against wrinkliness. The test will give us an absolute value for r as well as a p value. The value of r shows us the strength of association. (It varies between 0 and 1, with closest to 1 being strongest. It can be negative, indicating an inverse association, which would mean that in this example, as we age we get less wrinkly!) Statistical significance is said to be present by convention if a test gives a value of $p < 0.05$. What this means is that there is a less than 5% chance of the results shown in the study sample being by chance. If the tests were run again with samples from the same population, 95/100 the results would be the same. As we worked out in advance that the sample size was sufficient and our study was adequately powered (it had enough people in it to avoid errors), we can now say that as we age we get more wrinkly and that there is a strong correlation (as r = +0.990). We could also plot this on a scatter graph (Figure 7.5), and this plot would describe a line close to a left-to-right ascending diagonal line.

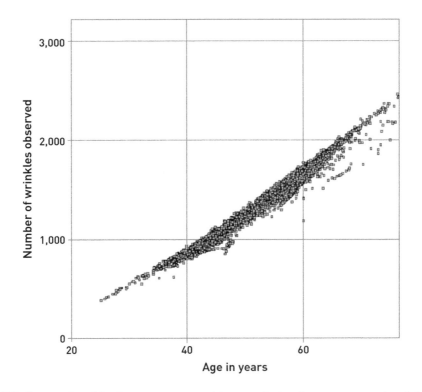

Figure 7.5: Scatterplot: this shows a strong positive correlation between age and wrinkles. Adapted from an original graph by Lars Aronsson (8 December 2008)

Next, we might decide to test our cream on different people. We assess the necessary sample size, recruit a random sample of people and then randomise them into a treatment and a control group. The treatment group will get our new cream, the control will get simple aqueous cream and the study will be double-blinded (neither researchers nor participants know whether they are getting the treatment or control cream). A baseline wrinkle measurement is taken at the start, participants are asked to use the creams for a month and then our investigators will reassess their wrinkles. We test the composition of each group at baseline to make sure that there were no biases in them; for example, if we had all the wrinkliest people in one group this would be a source of bias. At the end of the month we want to see if there are statistically significant differences between the groups, and this would be our hypothesis (the null hypothesis being that there are no differences between the groups; technically, then, we are trying to reject the null hypothesis to demonstrate that there are differences between groups).

We would use an unpaired or 'independent samples' t-test as the data are at ratio level, demonstrated (by us) to be normally distributed, and this test will compare means from each group (if we were able to compare data from each actual participant we could use a paired t-test). Using t-tests will give a value for the t-test and a p value, but the variables will be different from those mentioned above for correlations. In experimental designs, the independent variable will be the group into which participants are placed (treatment or control group creams) and the dependent variable will be the effect that each has on the wrinkles. So, in order to demonstrate that our new cream was effective, we would want to see a statistically significant difference (p < 0.05) between the two groups. If that was the case, we could report that the new cream was effective in reducing the numbers of wrinkles. We could also calculate CIs to give us the range of values of the means of the reduction in wrinkles in each group, and the size of this would indicate the relative accuracy of the results. For example, if the 95% CI for the treatment groups was 850–950 (this means that our measure of wrinkliness shows that the range is between 850 and 950 wrinkles per face) and the summary statistic was 900, this is a more accurate estimate than if the 95% CI for the control group was 500–2,500 wrinkles per face and the point estimate (or summary statistic) was 1,000.

We might think about being a bit more sophisticated with our analysis, and look at the impact that variables like age, sex, race, exposure to sunlight, location in the UK, smoking and so on might have on the outcomes of our study. In that case, as well as stratifying our sampling to reflect these properties at the outset, we could use an ANOVA technique, which would compare the means of these different variables and give us an indication of the relative importance of each. There are many different varieties of ANOVA, and we'd definitely want a statistician involved if we were planning to use one of these. Their advantage is that if we were to try to analyse each variable in a series of single comparisons, there is a danger of getting type I errors, as we would need to test so many times that occasionally one would occur by chance.

Assessing risk and clinical significance

Studies may or may not demonstrate statistical significance but this is a different concept to that of clinical significance. Risk can be assessed using epidemiological measures such as the relative risk (RR) and odds ratios (OR), which are used to describe the risk of contracting a disease. Number needed to treat (NNT) shows the clinical impact of treatment outcomes (Peat, 2002).

Relative risk

This describes associations between exposures and outcomes in prospective studies rather than case-controlled studies. It is quite a simple concept, where the rate of an illness in the exposed group is compared with that in the unexposed group. This could be used, for example, to show the RR to smokers of contracting lung cancer compared to non-smokers. It is time-dependent, as there are time factors associated with it, such as the time it takes to develop lung cancer (Peat, 2002). The results will be expressed by calculating CIs around a point estimate.

Odds ratios

These are not time-dependent and can be used in case-controlled studies where the proportions of cases and controls are limited because the sampling methods employed in the study mean that the prevalence of the disease in the study is not the same as the prevalence in the population. OR is similar to RR but not the same, and is calculated differently, giving the odds of contracting a disease. Thus the OR for contracting lung cancer if one is a smoker is different from the RR because the RR gives the risk of a person who is a smoker contracting lung cancer, while the OR shows the likelihood that a person with lung cancer has been a smoker. CIs around a point estimate will be calculated here too. If the range given by the CI includes 1.0 then the effect is not statistically significant, as 1.0 indicates that there is no RR or OR in one group compared to another (Peat, 2002). This is particularly useful if we have more than one factor involved in our analysis, as it can be drawn in a graph known as a forest plot (or 'blobbagram') and different results compared (Figure 7.6). It can also be used to compare and combine the results of individual studies (of which more in Chapter 8 on systematic reviews and meta-analyses).

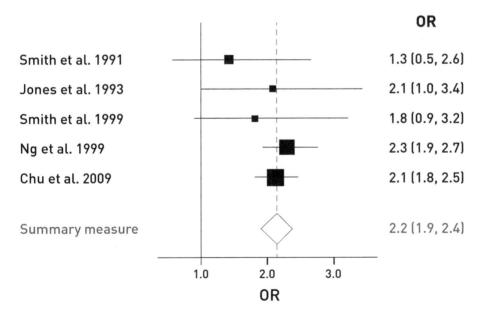

Figure 7.6: Forest plot: this shows confidence intervals, point estimates as black boxes and a summary measure in the larger diamond. OR, odds ratio. Reproduced from an original graph by Jimjamjak (4 May 2010)

In the example in Figure 7.6, to the left of the figure is the name of each individual study, the lines next to them are the CIs and the black boxes are the point estimates. You can see that in these studies Smith et al. (1991 and 1999) all overlap 1.0 so the effect is probably not statistically significant, even though the point estimate is greater than 1.0. Jones et al. (1993), Ng et al. (1999) and Chu et al. (2009) are less ambiguous as they do not cross 1.0. The overall odds ratio (the diamond) here is 2.0, meaning that the odds of having the disease in question (whatever it may be) are twice as great if a patient is exposed to some predisposing factor. (If Figure 7.6 represented smoking we could say that a patient with lung cancer is twice as likely, based on these studies, to be a smoker, but as the studies in this figure are not about lung cancer don't quote that!)

Number needed to treat

This can be calculated from randomised controlled trials and indicates how many patients would need to receive the new treatment for one additional patient to benefit (Peat, 2002). It allows for comparisons between treatments of their clinical effectiveness and cost-effectiveness, as a treatment that saves one additional life for every 10 patients treated is better than one that saves one additional life for every 100 patients treated. If they cost the same, then the first treatment is the most cost-effective. NNT is calculated by finding the absolute risk reduction (ARR) of each treatment and subtracting them (Peat, 2002). So, if one treatment reduces risk by 10% and another by 15%, 15 − 10 = 5% or 0.05 ARR. NNT = 1/ARR, or 1/0.05 = 20. This shows that 20 patients will need to take the new treatment to prevent one death. CIs would also be calculated for NNT.

Chapter summary

In this chapter we have explored approaches to quantitative data and offered some practical considerations on how to plan their analysis. We have introduced some basic concepts in statistics and statistical tests used in quantitative studies, and some ideas about how data can be presented and interpreted. We have looked at descriptive and inferential statistics, *p* values and CIs, RR, OR and NNT.

Activity answer

Activity 7.1: Research and finding evidence (page 121)

- Drinking alcohol: yes or no? Nominal data
- Number of alcoholic drinks consumed: Ratio data
- Satisfaction with the pub bar service: Ordinal data
- Number of men in the pub: Ratio data
- Number of women in the pub: Ratio data
- Income of each individual: Ratio data
- Pounds spent that evening: Ratio data
- Temperature in the bar area: Interval data

- Would return: yes or no? Nominal data
- Eating food: yes or no? Nominal data
- Satisfaction with the pub food service: Ordinal data

Further reading

Cullum, N, Ciliska, D, Haynes, RB and Marks, S (2008) *Evidence-Based Nursing: An Introduction.* Oxford: Blackwell Publishing.
Lots of relevant chapters on understanding and interpreting concepts discussed in this chapter.

De Vaus, DA (2002) *Surveys in Social Research,* 5th edition. London: Routledge.
Classic text on surveys that provides a good overview of the process.

Diamond, I and Jeffries, J (2001) *Beginning Statistics: An Introduction for Social Scientists.* London: Sage.

Background reading

Maltby, J, Day, L and Williams, G (2007) *Introduction to Statistics for Nurses.* Harlow: Pearson Education.
Very good background reading on statistics.

Parahoo, K (2006) *Nursing Research: Principles, Process and Issues,* 2nd edition. Basingstoke: Palgrave Macmillan.
Good, readable background information on study design and quantitative data analysis.

Peat, J (2002) *Health Science Research: A Handbook of Quantitative Methods, Part 6: Analysing the Data.* London: Sage.
Very good on the subject of which statistical tests to use and more depth than presented here.

Sapsford, R (2007) *Survey Research,* 2nd edition. London: Sage.
A readable and useful guide to survey research.

Useful websites

http://statpages.org
Web pages that perform statistical calculations from Statpages.org. Links and calculating pages.

www.ats.ucla.edu/stat/mult_pkg/whatstat/default.htm
University of California, Los Angeles guide to which statistics to use and how to run them in various computer packages.

www.medicine.ox.ac.uk/bandolier
Bandolier online evidence-based practice journal. Click on the Learning Zone link and then use the links on the left-hand side for more information about a range of topics discussed in this and the preceding chapter.

Chapter 8
Using and critiquing systematic reviews and meta-analyses

> **Chapter aims**
>
> After reading this chapter, you should be able to:
>
> - explain the rationale for systematic reviews and meta-analyses;
> - construct a protocol for a systematic review and meta-analysis;
> - understand which quantitative and qualitative techniques are used in meta-analysis;
> - explain the role of the Cochrane Collaboration and similar bodies;
> - describe how systematic reviews and meta-analyses inform the production of clinical guidelines and the work of NICE and SIGN.

Introduction

Having examined in previous chapters quantitative and qualitative research designs and their data analysis relating to single empirical studies, we will now move on to looking at how these can be amalgamated in systematic reviews (SRs) and meta-analyses. We are looking now at a secondary research technique, having spent much of the preceding pages looking at primary research studies and their designs. This is a comparatively recent development in nursing research, which has its roots in analysing experimental designs for medical decision making, and has now become an important global movement. It is essentially a simple idea: if lots of studies have been done in a broadly similar area, why not combine them and produce an overall result? SRs are a scientific research activity in themselves (Clarke, 2006), in which reviewers search out and include all papers relevant to a predefined question, and then combine them using statistical methods to produce a summary finding, like a 'headline', which is frequently a recommendation for healthcare decision making and/or changes in practice. Statistical techniques (for quantitative studies) or discussion (for qualitative work) give an overview (meta-analysis) of the key issues. Predefined questions are addressed using methodologies made explicit before the review starts, so that the studies discovered are included or excluded by relevant criteria so that any element of bias is ruled out (Clarke, 2006). Conversely one major flaw with *non-systematic* reviews is the extent to which researchers can include studies which give a biased picture of evidence that can be made to support their own views and so this systematic approach removes this (Hemingway and Brereton, 2009).

Rapid reviews, in which authors are commissioned to undertake a rapid assessment of the literature, making sure that 'users' (patients, clients, carers) are involved, are recent trends

(Hemingway and Brereton, 2009) which seek to make SRs relevant and responsive to changing healthcare demands.

The chapter begins by outlining the rationale for SRs and meta-analyses, and how to construct a protocol for an SR and meta-analysis. We will then go on to introduce some relevant quantitative and qualitative techniques. We will look at the work of the Cochrane Collaboration and other bodies, and then at how SRs and meta-analyses inform the production of clinical guidelines and the work of the National Institute for Health and Care Excellence (NICE) and other similar bodies.

Rationale for systematic reviews and meta-analyses

Mulrow (1995) outlines several key reasons why SRs are valuable as a scientific activity which aids healthcare decision making.

Rationale for systematic reviews, adapted from Mulrow (1995)

1. Large quantities of information are available in many healthcare fields and this needs to be condensed and refined into manageable units that can be explored critically and key findings need to be disseminated in an intelligible format.
2. As well as clinicians using SRs for decision making, researchers and policy makers use them for purposes such as economic evaluation, refining of hypotheses, sample sizes and variables.
3. Although time-consuming and exacting to carry out, SRs are usually cheaper and easier to undertake than large-scale studies that address and overcome flaws and limitations in previous studies. Updating SRs can lead to better understanding of issues as well as refining effect sizes. Mulrow (1995) quotes the example of streptokinase (a thrombolytic or clot-busting drug used to save lives post myocardial infarction) which, if relevant SRs had been updated as new studies became available, would have been shown to be effective 20 years earlier than when definitive evidence was available from primary studies.
4. Generalisability can be effectively assessed from SRs, as contextual information can be taken into account which can overcome the local context of studies that may have different eligibility criteria, disease definitions and study designs.
5. Consistency of relationships can be established. SRs can show that findings from several studies point in the same direction. In experimental designs, the magnitude and direction of treatments can be indicated, whereas in qualitative studies a narrative can be constructed which indicates the overall themes from each study. Similarly, SRs can also indicate inconsistencies and conflicts in the data.
6. Quantitative SRs can establish power and precision, meaning that the statistical analyses from several studies can be combined to give a more authoritative

statistical meta-analysis when the studies are pooled, and estimates of effect sizes can become more precise. We will examine how this is done in more detail later.

7. Accuracy: by using explicit scientific principles for the inclusion and exclusion of studies, SRs overcome the potential bias associated with non-systematic reviews, which is the danger that researchers include evidence that only supports their own theoretical position.

In addition, Hemingway and Brereton (2009) add that SRs can give authoritative 'headline' findings for use in healthcare decision making; are increasingly a requirement of undergraduate and postgraduate research work; and are central to the NICE health technology assessment process for technology appraisals and the production of clinical guidelines.

Writing a proposal for a systematic review

A proposal for an SR is usually known as a protocol. While most institutions will want you to write a proposal for an empirical primary research study, some may allow you to construct an SR instead.

Khan et al. (2003) outline a five-stage approach:

1. framing questions for a review;
2. identifying relevant literature;
3. assessing the quality of the literature;
4. summarising the evidence;
5. interpreting the findings.

Stage 1: Framing questions for a review

Rather than PICO, which we looked at in Chapter 2, Khan et al. (2003) use the mnemonic PIOS – population, intervention (or exposure), outcomes and study designs (suitable for addressing the questions). This will allow you to design a structured question as well as indicate which types of study design are suitable for answering your question. Questions asking for information on 'what works best' are likely to be answered by experimental designs, whereas questions asking 'what are patients' experience of illness?' are likely to be best answered by qualitative designs.

Stage 2: Identifying relevant literature

We have already discussed issues in literature searching. In an SR protocol, you must show that you plan to be thorough and exhaustive, and present a review plan that is free from bias and transparent in being able to find everything that has been published in an area. You will want to outline a large number of search terms, exploring the topic from many different angles, as well as listing all the databases you will search and including Cochrane and NICE guidelines. You should have a plan for dealing with grey literature (unpublished material, conference presentations that are not published as articles, PhD theses) and be ready to e-mail authors and scour reference lists for material not identified in other ways. You need to reconcile sensitivity with precision: a review that is 100% sensitive to every possible paper is likely to be quite imprecise and so you are likely to get lots of papers not directly relevant to the subject. A precise search may run the risk of missing papers which do not exactly fit the search terms but will give you a smaller number of papers to review. Publication bias is also an issue: smaller studies or studies with non-significant results are less likely to be published, so it is possible that studies you find, when meta-analysed, overestimate the extent to which the new treatment or intervention is effective. Once you have searched your databases using multiple search terms, you will need to apply inclusion and exclusion criteria, and these should be stated in advance. This extraction of papers is crucial to getting appropriate evidence and is known as screening.

Stage 3: Assessing the quality of the literature

Critiquing research reports and giving a critical appraisal of a body of literature are large topics in themselves. In a protocol you should outline what criteria are to be used. It is unlikely that you'll develop these yourself, and appropriate frameworks such as those given on the NHS Critical Appraisal Skills Programme (CASP) website (http://www.casp-uk.net) will be useful for you. More than one person should independently screen and review the retrieved searches as an additional step in rigour in SRs. The quality of studies is frequently assessed and given numerical values based on the criteria employed. Reviewers should agree a cut-off point for inclusion of studies and discuss and agree independently which ones should be included and why. A summary of the papers included and excluded and the criteria used should be given: a useful tool for showing this is the flow diagram from PRISMA (http://www.prisma-statement. org) which can be downloaded as a Word document.

Stage 4: Summarising the evidence

We discuss issues in meta-analyses in qualitative, quantitative and mixed method SRs in more detail below. In your protocol you should outline exactly how this will be done, including some reference to the relative heterogeneity and how it might be tested (in quantitative reviews) or otherwise accounted for (in qualitative ones). In all reviews, but particularly in mixed method ones, you may also have methodological heterogeneity (Khan et al., 2003). This may make combining studies difficult, but their findings can still be contrasted and assessed.

Stage 5: Interpreting the findings

If you are writing a protocol, you won't have any interpretation to do, but the key issues are as follows (Khan et al., 2003):

- Are the searches adequate? Is it clear that the search has been thorough, transparent and free from bias?

- Are there publication biases? Funnel plots can be used to indicate publication bias.
- Is the quality of the included studies high enough? This will be derived from your critical appraisal of the included studies. It may be that the quality of the studies is such that they cannot be meta-analysed.
- Are any outcomes clinically significant? Are changes in policy and practice necessary, and are new approaches to research required?

While the processes of systematically searching, including/excluding papers and reviewing the literature are broadly similar, quantitative and qualitative techniques, meta-analysis and synthesis of the literature are quite different. We will now go on to examine these key differences.

Quantitative systematic reviews and meta-analyses

If the initial research question is about 'What works best?' and there are clear comparisons between an active treatment (or intervention) and a control (or usual care), then study designs in the papers retrieved will include experimental, quasi-experimental and cohort studies. The aims of meta-analysis in this case are to estimate an overall effect size and whether the effect is roughly similar or dissimilar in different settings. This can be summarised in a narrative form if the papers are relatively heterogeneous (dissimilar), meaning that the papers are discussed rather than statistically analysed (NHS Centre for Reviews and Dissemination (NHS CRD), 2006). If the studies are relatively homogeneous (similar), they can be combined statistically. If possible the measurements used in the studies can be used to pool their results, and usually this is presented for an intervention as the extent to which change was affected. This is presented differently if the data are in binary or continuous form. Odds ratios can be used if the data are binary, but these can overestimate treatment effects. Differences in means or standardised mean differences (d-statistics, z-scores and effect sizes) are used if the data are continuous (NHS CRD, 2006).

Results are usually presented in a forest plot (so called because it can look a bit like a tree). If we turn back to Figure 7.6 (page 132), where we looked at how odds ratios are presented, the format of this figure is similar to the presentation of statistical meta-analysis. For the purposes of meta-analysis, however, the line 1.0 is used to assess the effectiveness of treatment, so studies to the left of 1.0 on the graph indicate that the active treatment is better, whereas those to the right of the line indicate that the active treatment is worse. In Figure 7.6 we can also see that the studies have received a weighting, and this is represented by how large the effect size box is drawn. We can see that Jones et al. (1993, 1999) have relatively small effect sizes whereas Ng et al. (1999) and Chu et al. (2009) have much bigger boxes. This weighting takes into account the relative size of the study, with the largest studies receiving the largest weighting. So we can see that, as 1.0 = no difference between the active or control groups, and the summary effect size diamond = 2.0, the active treatment is worse than the control in this example.

Fixed and random effects models

Fixed effects models ignore the studies' heterogeneity and assume that the treatment effects are consistent across studies. Random effects models assume that other factors may modify treatment effects, are usually more conservative in their estimation of confidence intervals and can give too much weight to smaller studies, whereas fixed effects models may produce too precise treatment effects. Methods used in each are Mantel–Haenszel and Peto odds ratios, and means for fixed effects models; random effect models use DerSimonian and Laird, and Bayesian models. These are quite complex terms and you are not expected to do much more at this level than recognise them as types of tests used in statistical meta-analysis. More information can be found in NHS CRD (2006).

Studies in a review can also be tested for heterogeneity, publication bias (using funnel plots) and sensitivity using sensitivity analysis: the latter indicates how robust the overall analysis is (NHS CRD, 2006). Testing for heterogeneity is important because, if the studies are too dissimilar, reviewers run the risk of combining things that are not alike. For example, if one trial used a new analgesic in only the postoperative period, should its findings be amalgamated with one in which the analgesic was continued for three months? If the first study used it in a dosage of 30 mg twice daily, can it be meta-analysed with one where 60 mg four times daily was used? What if the studies used different pain-scoring techniques? There are statistical tests used in testing for heterogeneity, including chi-squared and the I statistic. Authors should investigate heterogeneity and it should be reported; if not it is a serious limitation. If the studies retrieved are simply too dissimilar and statistical analysis is meaningless, then they can still be synthesised but the authors would need to discuss their results in a written rather than statistical form, known as narrative synthesis.

Publication bias is slightly more difficult to establish. In general, positive studies (studies that show something) are more likely to be published, even though non-statistically significant results may be just as clinically important as statistically significant ones. This means that, if a literature search and subsequent meta-analysis were carried out, it would overstate the extent to which any new treatment or intervention had positive results. In theory, it should be possible to plot the results of each study in the review on a graph, and it should look like a pyramid (or funnel). If there is a bite or chunk missing from the funnel, this could indicate publication bias. In Figure 8.1, you can see a funnel plot with a good, nearly symmetrical spread of data. The points represent results in studies found by the reviewers. On the x (horizontal) axis would be the result statistics (for example, risk ratios) and on the y (vertical) axis would be sample size. In Figure 8.2 you can see the funnel plot redrawn with some of the small, inconclusive or negative results omitted, as if the reviewers had not found them because they had not been published (or even suppressed). You can see in Figure 8.2 that there is a chunk missing, so the funnel plot is asymmetrical, indicating possible publication bias. Publication bias demonstrated like this might be something of a tentative finding because it may be that actually there are no studies to find (Gough et al., 2012).

Authors of SRs may show funnel plots, and should also convince you that they have gone to great lengths to find all possible studies, including unpublished studies, to overcome possible publication bias and make sure their meta-analysis conclusions are based on the widest available evidence.

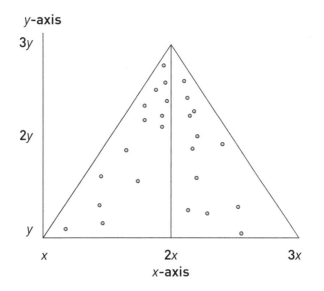

Figure 8.1: Generic funnel plot. Reproduced from an original graph by Nousernamesleft (21 January 2008). Made freely available for any purpose under the Wikimedia Creative Commons License via Wikipedia (see http://commons.wikimedia.org/wiki/Main_Page for further information)

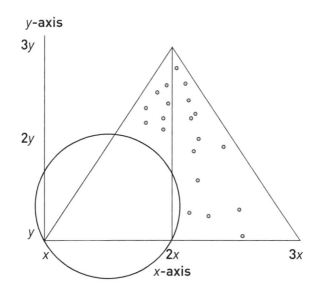

Figure 8.2: Funnel plot showing publication bias. Adapted from an original graph by Nousernamesleft (21 January 2008). Made freely available for any purpose under the Wikimedia Creative Commons License via Wikipedia (see http://commons.wikimedia.org/wiki/Main_Page for further information)

Sensitivity analysis in a quantitative SR can be tested by removing the results of one or more studies from the analysis to examine the impact that this has on the meta-analysis. If there are a small number of studies, the overall synthesis might be dominated by one or two, so removing them can illustrate if this is the case and allow the reviewers to make judgements about the robustness of their analysis (Gough et al., 2012).

Qualitative systematic reviews and meta-analyses

As there has been a large growth in qualitative research in recent years, techniques have been developed which allow overviews of these studies to be constructed. While searching, including and reviewing studies will be similar processes, there can be no statistical meta-analysis as there would be with experimental designs. This leads qualitative searchers to use different terminology for their meta-analysis, and terms such as meta-study and meta-synthesis are used instead, as is the term meta-ethnography (Lloyd Jones, 2006). Some qualitative reviews will be largely descriptive, but generally they are interpretative in that they seek to synthesise a number of studies' findings and reinterpret them to give an overview of the body of literature and offer new insights and understandings which can provide a foundation for future research and advance thinking about key issues (Lloyd Jones, 2006).

One common criticism of qualitative research is that it does not produce generalisable findings, so it is much more difficult for the meaning of qualitative studies to be interpreted in different settings. However, if several qualitative studies could be combined, then the similarities and differences of the primary studies could be used to inform research and practice in that field. The rich, indepth data gained from patients and service users is useful to understand patients' experiences of illness, service delivery and barriers to service usage (Ring et al., 2011) and so synthesis of qualitative studies is important.

Unlike quantitative meta-analysis, which can be accomplished in a relatively straightforward statistical manner if the studies are homogeneous, qualitative evidence synthesis is more tentative, exploratory and contested. This is an emerging field and there are a variety of different ways in which it can be done. Unless they take a generic qualitative approach, qualitative studies will have particular philosophical perspectives, and are very much derived from the context and subjective views of participants (Ring et al., 2011), meaning that one group of participants may give quite different views than another because their experiences might be entirely dissimilar. This does not mean that there is something wrong with qualitative research studies with conflicting findings, just that human beings can experience any aspect of the world very differently.

Although searching for studies ought to be as rigorous a process as in a quantitative SR, quality appraisal of qualitative studies is not straightforward and there is little consensus about what the criteria might be for high-quality qualitative studies (Ring et al., 2011).

It is beyond the scope of this book to detail the similarities and differences between qualitative evidence synthesis techniques; Ring et al. (2011) list the following methods:

- critical interpretive synthesis;
- grounded theory synthesis;
- meta-ethnography;
- meta-interpretation;
- meta-study;
- meta-summary;

- qualitative cross-case analysis;
- thematic synthesis.

In qualitative evidence synthesis, results are interpreted by reviewers. The studies may be quite different in their settings and contexts, but novel conceptualisations and extrapolations are drawn that go beyond the studies included (Lloyd Jones, 2006). Key features are outlined in the box below.

Key features of a meta-synthesis

Lloyd Jones (2006) gives the following as key features of a meta-synthesis:

1. Focus of study, inclusion and exclusion criteria and theoretical framework: rather than having a 'what works best?' question, the focus may be on broad areas or concepts, and may also be meaningful and relevant for healthcare decision making. Inclusion criteria may be about samples, settings and themes, and possibly methodologies.
2. Study identification: this will be by an exhaustive literature search, in the same way that any other review would be undertaken.
3. Study selection: this is a less precise field than in statistical meta-analysis, given that less precise criteria are used to assess the quality of qualitative studies. Once again, precision must be reconciled with sensitivity in the search.
4. Summary analysis and synthesis of findings: findings can be synthesised using formal techniques such as grounded formal theory and meta-ethnography, but less structured approaches of interpretation can also be used. Whichever methods are used should be clearly specified and transparent, with categories developed similar to themes and subthemes in primary studies, with an eye on uniqueness for emerging theories and evidence which confirms and refutes them. Lots of different ways of analysing the data should be considered, and tabulation is important, meaning that the studies included should be grouped together in a table showing which themes are shared, confirmed and refuted by using which studies. Date, geography, methodology and other categories can also be used to tabulate findings, but interpretations must be based on themes or theories that emerge rather than these already-existing categories.
5. Interpretation of results: this will depend on the field and initial question(s) and reviewers will need to tailor their work to their audiences.

Combining mixed methods studies in a systematic review

If a review is not driven by a clear 'what works?' question, it is likely that studies from multiple methodologies may be obtained. This will necessitate their review and meta-analysis using a combination of approaches, outlined above. This means that the interpretation will be more complex, but it is possible to compare findings of the different meta-analysis methods and use the insights gained from the different methodological approaches to triangulate the results of the review.

Cochrane Collaboration and other bodies

The Cochrane Collaboration

The Cochrane Collaboration (www.cochrane.org) is named after Archie Cochrane, an epidemiologist who pioneered the use of randomised controlled trials as a means of informing healthcare practice. It is an independent, not-for-profit organisation and receives funding from various sources, including governments, universities, hospital trusts, charities and personal donations. It was established in 1993 as an international network and makes freely accessible Cochrane Reviews via its Library, which is searchable, free of charge.

Figure 8.3 is the logo of the Cochrane Collaboration. It incorporates a forest plot showing the meta-analysis of the use of corticosteroids with pregnant women to improve outcomes for their premature babies. The meta-analysis indicates that steroid usage improves outcomes, as the summary (the diamond) is to the left of the line. Outcomes were 30–50% better when the mothers had been treated before birth with steroids. Changes in practice have resulted from this meta-analysis as it provides clear evidence of the clinical effectiveness of the treatment.

The Joanna Briggs Institute

The Joanna Briggs Institute (http://joannabriggs.org) is an international, not-for-profit research and development organisation within the Faculty of Health Sciences at the

Figure 8.3: The Cochrane Collaboration logo. Used with permission from Nick Royle, CEO, the Cochrane Collaboration, Oxford, UK

University of Adelaide. It makes accessible resources for evidence-based healthcare for nurses, midwives, medics and allied health professionals. It seeks to improve the health status of the global population through the delivery of evidence-based healthcare. This is achieved by developing methods to appraise and synthesise evidence and by conducting SRs and analyses of the research literature, as well as dissemination and implementation of evidence.

The Cochrane Nursing Care Field

The Cochrane Nursing Care Field (http://cncf.cochrane.org/home) was established in 2009 as a result of the initiative of nurses at the Joanna Briggs Institute in Australia. It has three functions related to the production and use of Cochrane reviews, which are: to support Cochrane in the preparation of reviews relevant to nursing; to introduce perspectives relevant to all those providing nursing care (nurses, other disciplines such as social work, families and lay caregivers); and to enhance the dissemination and effective uptake of Cochrane reviews.

NHS Institute for Health Research Centre for Reviews and Dissemination (CRD)

The CRD (www.york.ac.uk/inst/crd) is a department of the University of York and is part of the National Institute for Health Research. It is responsible for undertaking high-quality SRs to evaluate the effects of health and social care interventions and the delivery and organisation of healthcare.

Database of Abstracts of Reviews of Effects (DARE)

DARE contains 15,000 abstracts of SRs, including over 6,000 quality-assessed reviews, as well as details of all Cochrane reviews and protocols.

NHS Economic Evaluation Database (EED)

NHS EED contains 24,000 abstracts of health economics papers, including over 7,000 quality-assessed economic evaluations. It is aimed at decision makers and identifies, describes and appraises economic evaluations.

Health Technology Assessment (HTA) database

The HTA database brings together and describes details of completed and ongoing health technology assessments from around the world.

NHS Evidence

NHS Evidence (www.evidence.nhs.uk/default.aspx) includes more than 150 sources, including internationally respected evidence-based sources such as the Cochrane Library, *British*

National Formulary and Map of Medicine. Resources available include guidelines, drug information, primary research and clinical summaries.

Activity 8.1   *Research and finding evidence, and critical thinking*

This is likely to be a time-consuming activity and may need to be revisited and refined over a number of days, particularly in terms of your search questions, which is why there is only one activity in this chapter! Don't print the studies you find, just read the abstracts on screen. You can save the abstracts to a folder in your computer and return to them later on.

1. Using Khan et al.'s (2003) mnemonic PIOS (population, intervention, outcomes, study design), produce a question for yourself based on your clinical nursing interests.
2. Search all the databases given immediately above and write a list of the reviews you find. How many have you found? Are they similar? Are they the same reviews? Do they have similar findings and recommendations? How do these reviews compare to current practice in your area?
3. Next, frame the question differently so that it contains the phrase 'patients' experiences of'. Use your university library journal search database and Google Scholar. What kinds of papers are identified now? Ask yourself the same questions as in point 2, above. How do the results from these two sets of searches compare? Are there differences between the qualitative and quantitative literature?
4. Write a short synthesis of findings from each search. Is one methodology overwhelmingly represented in your results? Are there flaws you can identify in any of the studies? Are there consistencies or inconsistencies in the recommendations from each methodology? Are changes in practice required in your area?

This represents your assessment of this body of literature, so there is no answer at the end of the chapter.

How systematic reviews and meta-analyses inform the production of clinical guidelines
NICE and SIGN

NICE (www.nice.org.uk) provides guidance, sets quality standards and manages a national database to improve people's health and prevent and treat ill health. There is a searchable database on the website. NICE makes recommendations on:

- new and existing medicines, treatments and procedures;
- treating and caring for people with specific diseases and conditions;
- how to improve people's health and prevent illness and disease.

These recommendations from NICE guidelines are not compulsory, but they are a key aspect of standard setting and clinical governance throughout the NHS. NICE also works towards implementation and has specific implementation activities and plans to make sure research findings change practice.

The Scottish Intercollegiate Guidelines Network (SIGN: www.sign.ac.uk) undertakes similar activities for the NHS in Scotland. It commissions reviews of the literature and produces guidelines for Scotland with the aim of improving Scottish health, reducing variations in care and disseminating best practice. There are broad similarities between NICE and SIGN (outlined at http://www.sign.ac.uk/about/niceandsign.html).

NICE and SIGN use similar processes to an SR and meta-analysis to form conclusions and recommendations on particular clinical questions. An exhaustive search is carried out, studies are tabulated and their quality assessed. Various methods of assessment can be used. It is common that papers will be judged using some form of hierarchy of evidence, as this means that different types of research and evidence can be given a weighting to indicate their importance, and the overall quality of the evidence assessed. In this, the clinical effectiveness of different study designs is assessed and those higher in the hierarchy gain greater weight. You'll see many different formulations of hierarchies of evidence, but all are reasonably similar. The one shown in Table 8.1 has been adapted from the University of Oxford Centre for Evidence Based Medicine (CEBM: www.cebm.net) and relates to therapeutic interventions.

Level	Study design
1a	Systematic reviews and meta-analyses of randomised controlled trials (with homogeneity)
1b	Individual randomised controlled trials with narrow confidence intervals
2a	Systematic reviews and meta-analyses of cohort studies* (with homogeneity)
2b	Individual cohort study
3a	Systematic reviews and meta-analyses of case-controlled studies† (with homogeneity)
3b	Individual case-controlled studies
4	Case series‡ or poor cohort or case-controlled studies
5	Expert opinion

Table 8.1: Centre for Evidence Based Medicine hierarchy of evidence (adapted from Howick, 2009)

* A cohort study is one in which one group of patients received an intervention and another did not, and they are followed to assess the outcomes. This is a pragmatic design and patients are not recruited or randomised by the researchers.

† A case-controlled study is one in which patients are identified by outcome and compared to others without that outcome to assess whether they had the same exposure.

‡ A case series study is one where patients are assessed for outcomes without a control or comparison group.

If this hierarchy was used for grading a body of literature and to make recommendations, as is frequently the case in NICE and SIGN guidelines, it would produce a grading strategy which looks like the one in Table 8.2. A set of guidelines with mostly grade A studies would have a robust evidence base and be suitable for recommending changes to clinical practice.

Grade	Assessment
A	Mostly level 1 studies
B	Consistently level 2 or 3 studies
C	Level 4 studies
D	Level 5 studies or inconsistent or inconclusive studies at any level

Table 8.2: Grading structure for recommendations (adapted from Howick, 2009)

This CEBM definition does not include any qualitative research in its assessment of the effectiveness of different study designs. Some authors publish hierarchies of evidence which include qualitative studies; for example, Moule and Goodman (2009) present and discuss a model adapted from various sources which shows qualitative work as rating at level 4 in a hierarchy of evidence. Daly et al. (2007) propose a separate hierarchy for qualitative work (Table 8.3), although this is yet to be widely accepted by bodies such as NICE and SIGN.

Level	Study design
I	Generalisable studies*
II	Conceptual studies†
III	Descriptive studies‡
IV	Single-case studies§

Table 8.3: Hierarchy of evidence for qualitative work (adapted from Daly et al., 2007)

* Generalisable studies are those with an extensive literature review which build on strong theoretical and methodological frameworks.
† Conceptual studies are those where a clear conceptual framework developed from previous studies guides sampling and analysis.
‡ Descriptive studies are those which may be atheoretical and focus on sampling from a particular location or group.
§ Single-case studies are those which provide data from one or a very small number of participants.

Daly et al.'s (2007) ideas are controversial in that many qualitative researchers would strongly dispute the relevance of the concept of generalisability in relation to their work. Quantitative researchers and those conducting randomised controlled trials might also argue that it is impossible to tell the impact or effectiveness of most qualitative studies as they contain no measurements, but this is to reopen well-rehearsed arguments which we were at pains to move beyond in Chapter 1.

NICE and SIGN guidelines can also use an adaptation of an assessment known as GRADE (Grading of Recommendations Assessment, Development and Evaluation), which is an approach to assessing the quality of evidence (NICE, 2009). Recommendations are then constructed by a review panel in which many aspects of the literature include clinical- and cost-effectiveness. The recommendations may be indicated as strong to weak, where strong recommendations are a product of a high-quality evidence base.

National Service Frameworks

As well as NICE and SIGN guidance, the NHS has also produced National Service Frameworks (NSFs) which set out standards and expectations within which NHS services must operate. They were constructed in consultation with patients, carers and professionals, as well as with robust assessment of the available research evidence. A full list of NSFs is given on the NHS Choices website (www.nhs.uk/nhsengland/nsf/pages/nationalserviceframeworks.aspx). They use a similar grading strategy to that outlined above, which allows different weightings to be given to different types of evidence. The NSF for Older People (Department of Health, 2001, page 17/202) does include qualitative research in its typology, at level B3 (on an eight-point scale from A1 to D), specifying that they must be well designed.

Criticisms of systematic reviews and meta-analyses

SRs are not without their critics, however. The eminent psychologist Eysenck (1995) outlines some criticisms in the box below.

Criticisms of systematic reviews, adapted from Eysenck (1995)

1. Including all possible studies means just that: everything – good, bad and indifferent – is included, and so the exemplary studies and their estimation of treatment effects can be corrupted by poorer work. Rather, it would be more useful to look for inconsistencies and anomalies in the data.
2. Meta-analyses give simplified answers that do not take into account the interplay of multiple variables and reducing the coverage of material included in reviews makes it difficult to consider explanations which do not appear in the included studies.
3. Meta-analysis is only meaningful if there is a high degree of homogeneity, that is, if the studies are relatively similar, and if they are relatively dissimilar (heterogeneous) their combination is difficult, if not meaningless.

Eysenck (1995, page 73) concludes by saying that if a medical treatment had an effect so recondite (difficult to understand) and obscure as to require meta-analysis to establish it, he would not be happy to have it used on him. However, it is fair to say that the science of meta-analysis has moved on considerably since he wrote this, and evidence-based or informed decision making is now established as a global strategy for improving healthcare practice.

Critiquing a systematic review and meta-analysis

Although SRs published by Cochrane are likely to be exhaustive and authoritative, not all SRs in all journals will be as good. It is possible that you may find considerably poorer ones. CASP provides a tool for critiquing SRs and meta-analyses (http://www.casp-uk.net). Hemingway and Brereton (2009) list the following as essential issues in ascertaining the quality of an SR and meta-analysis paper:

1. Is the topic well defined? Is there a clear and clinically relevant question which the reviewers seek to answer?
2. Was the search for papers thorough?
3. Were the criteria for inclusion applied fairly and consistently?
4. Was quality assessed independently by reviewers?
5. Was any missing information sought from authors?
6. Do the included studies indicate similar effects? If not, has heterogeneity been assessed?
7. Are the overall findings robust? Has publication bias been addressed?
8. Has the impact of chance been addressed? If there are few studies with statistically significant findings, does that indicate flaws in the studies, or gaps in the literature, or is there really nothing known about the question?
9. Are the recommendations clearly based on the evidence from the review? Or has any element of bias been introduced by reviewers?

Chapter summary

In this chapter, we began by outlining the rationale for SRs and meta-analyses. This was that there are vast quantities of research evidence available, and techniques have been developed to synthesise these so that results from many studies can be viewed as a whole to provide useful overviews for healthcare decision making. We then looked at how to construct a protocol for an SR and meta-analysis, making the point that these include thorough and exhaustive literature searching and appraisal of the evidence. Next, we introduced relevant quantitative and qualitative techniques used in meta-analysis, before moving on to talk about the Cochrane Collaboration, and how SRs and meta-analyses inform the production of clinical guidelines and the work of NICE and SIGN.

Further reading

Britten, N, Campbell, R, Pope, C, Donovan, J, Morgan, M and Pill, R (2002) Using meta-ethnography to synthesise qualitative research: a worked example. *Journal of Health Services Research and Policy*, 7 (4): 209–215.
Some further insights into using meta-ethnography to synthesise qualitative research.

Crombie, IK and Davies, HTO (2009) *What Is Meta Analysis? Bandolier Evidence Based Medicine Series.* Available online at www.medicine.ox.ac.uk/bandolier/painres/download/whatis/Meta-An.pdf. This is particularly relevant to issues in this chapter.

Garside, R, Britten, N and Stein, K (2008) The experience of heavy menstrual bleeding: a systematic review and meta-ethnography of qualitative studies. *Journal of Advanced Nursing*, 63 (6): 550–562.
An example of a qualitative systematic review.

Gough, D, Oliver, S and Thomas, J (2012) *An Introduction to Systematic Reviews.* London: Sage.
A good introduction by authors from the EPPI-Centre for Systematic Reviews (see Useful websites, below).

Greenhalgh, T (1997) How to read a paper: papers that summarise other papers (systematic reviews and meta-analyses). *British Medical Journal*, 315: 672–675.
Classic paper on this area.

Heyvaert, M, Maes, B and Onghena, P (2013) Mixed methods research synthesis: definition, framework, and potential. *Quality & Quantity*, 47 (2): 659–676.

Higgins, JTP, Thompson, SG, Deeks, JJ and Altman, DG (2003) Measuring inconsistency in meta-analyses. *British Medical Journal*, 327 (7414): 557–560. Available online at http://www.ncbi.nlm.nih.gov/pmc/articles/PMC192859.

Sandelowski, M and Barroso, J (2007) *Handbook for Synthesising Qualitative Research.* New York: Springer.

Souza, JP, Pileggi, C and Cecatti, JG (2007) Assessment of funnel plot asymmetry and publication bias in reproductive health meta-analyses: an analytic survey. *Reproductive Health*, 4: 3.
This study looks at publication bias in systematic reviews and meta-analyses in reproductive research.

Webb, C and Roe, B (2006) *Reviewing Research Evidence for Nursing Practice: Systematic Reviews.* Oxford: Blackwell.
Lots of good examples of qualitative systematic reviews.

Useful websites

http://eppi.ioe.ac.uk/cms
The Evidence for Policy and Practice Information and Co-ordinating Centre (EPPI-Centre) is part of the Social Science Research Unit at the Institute of Education, University of London. They conduct systematic reviews and develop methodological aspects.

http://www.prisma-statement.org
PRISMA (Preferred Reporting Items for Systematic Reviews and Meta-Analyses) provides an evidence-based minimum set of items for reporting in systematic reviews and meta-analyses.

http://www.youtube.com/user/UABEBMcourse?feature=watch
Terry Shaneyfelt from the University of Alabama Birmingham School of Medicine has an excellent series of short videos on YouTube covering many aspects of quantitative meta-analysis and topics related to systematic reviews.

www.medicine.ox.ac.uk/bandolier/learnzone.html
Bandolier Learning Zone. Contains lots of relevant materials on these and other topics.

Section 4
Writing and finishing

Chapter 9
Writing up your literature review and documentary analysis

Chapter aims

After reading this chapter, you should be able to:

- structure and write up a literature review;
- organise your references in a systematic manner;
- analyse and write a documentary analysis;
- understand how to use content analysis, and what the advantages and disadvantages of this approach might be.

Introduction

Section 4 includes two chapters focusing on the final stage of writing up. In this chapter, we guide you through the process of structuring and writing up your literature review or documentary analysis. This will include understanding the purpose of your literature review, identifying the different structures that can be used and appreciating the importance of being thorough and systematic. We will also examine how to analyse and write up a documentary analysis. A specific approach to analysing documentary data, content analysis, will be outlined and the strengths and weaknesses of this approach will be discussed.

In Chapter 10, we will introduce you to some basic writing skills and give you some tips about how to structure and write your research proposal or dissertation. We will examine what barriers you may experience to the writing process and we will stress the importance of writing as soon as possible rather than waiting until the later stages of your project.

Writing up your literature review

In this chapter, we outline how to write up your literature review, either as a stand-alone piece of work or as part of an empirical research study. This builds upon Chapter 2, where you were introduced to the process of undertaking a literature search to identify the key literature for your research topic.

Your literature review needs to be thorough and systematic to ensure that it does not cover only the literature that supports your beliefs and therefore ignores any material that may challenge them. Indeed, the literature that challenges your beliefs can be your most valuable resource because it makes you question and explore your viewpoint.

There are a number of key elements to a literature review and the emphasis that you give to each component depends upon your individual project. The key elements are:

- definitions for the key terminology you will use;
- the historical background to your research topic and the current context of your research topic, demonstrating how it is important and relevant;
- a discussion of relevant concepts and theories that you will use;
- a critical evaluation of previous studies, addressing their strengths and weaknesses and any gaps that have not been addressed;
- if you are undertaking empirical data collection, it also enables you to justify how your research will extend or challenge previous studies or respond to a gap in your field.

Your literature review should provide a coherent and critical account of the literature, identifying patterns and themes as well as evaluating the quality of the material. One of the features of a good literature review is that it acknowledges that most topics are contested terrain in which competing viewpoints are expressed. This means that you need to provide an active account that evaluates the available evidence and demonstrates your own voice as an author, rather than a passive description of these different accounts.

Case study: The opening paragraph

In Chapter 2, you were introduced to Sarah, a student on a mental health placement. Sarah is interested in how the media portrays women with a diagnosis of schizophrenia and has decided to use documentary analysis for her research project within a feminist paradigm. She is writing up her literature review and has written the following paragraph:

Bhutto (2008) found that news stories in newspapers were more likely to use discriminatory language than the same news story on television. Jones (2005) argues that tabloid newspapers are the major source of discriminatory accounts of women with mental health problems. Begum (2001) found that, although television reports did use discriminatory language, this was not as often as in newspaper accounts.

Activity 9.1   *Critical thinking*

What are the weaknesses in this paragraph? What improvements might you recommend to Sarah?

There is a brief summary of answers and a suggested alternative paragraph at the end of the chapter.

The key message is that you need to avoid a 'shopping list' approach, in which you provide an inventory of previous research studies without an overall narrative. As well as evaluating the quality of individual studies, your analysis should make links between studies, highlighting similarities and differences and drawing out the main issues.

A good literature review will not take what has previously been written at face value but will be aware of the contested nature of knowledge, in which alternative views and positions may be taken. It will also be sensitive to issues of power, where some viewpoints are privileged while others are marginalised.

Structuring your literature review

You need to have a clear overall structure to your literature review and there are a number of different options. One option is a chronological structure, looking at how your research topic has been written about over a period of time. This is particularly useful when your research topic shows a clear historical development. For example, a literature review of patient involvement could use a specific time period and discuss how public attitudes towards health services have developed from a paternalistic model to expectations that patients are more involved in decisions about their care. Another alternative is to structure your literature review thematically, focusing on what concepts or theoretical models are addressed. Using the same example, the literature review could be structured according to the different philosophies that underpin patient involvement (managerialist versus emancipatory models) or the sites of involvement (staff recruitment, service planning and training).

A general concept used to describe the structure of literature reviews is *funnelling*. This describes a process in which the literature review begins with a broad discussion that aims to provide a backdrop or background context for the research and there is a progressive narrowing of the focus. This can be achieved in a number of ways and some commonly used structures are as follows:

- Moving from the most general literature to that which is most closely related to your work. For example, briefly discussing the wider literature in your field, focusing more on some of the literature in your general topic area but saving your most detailed analysis for the research that is closest to your research topic.
- A chronological structure, moving from the earliest literature to the most recent.
- A 'compare and contrast' or dialectical approach, in which you outline one approach, contrast it with a second approach and then introduce a third approach (Weissberg and Buker, 1990, pages 45–46).

When you are preparing the outline of your literature review, it can be helpful to write a detailed argument structure. This is the series of steps that you will follow in developing your argument and enables you to establish quickly whether it has a logical progression. For example, if you were writing a literature review about bereavement using a chronological structure, your argument structure might look something like this:

1. Introduction to the concept of bereavement, including definitions.
2. Chronological review of bereavement models, such as Kübler-Ross (1970) and her stage model.

3. Critical appraisal of Kübler-Ross's model (e.g. seen as overly prescriptive with insufficient weight given to social context).
4. Discussion of more recent models of bereavement and how they address shortcomings of earlier models; for example, Walter's (1996) 'new model of grief', which focuses on sociological concepts of identity and argues that the purpose of grief is to sustain the link with the lost person rather than to 'move on'.
5. Conclusion – review of developments in models of bereavement.

Try to avoid overly relying upon headings to communicate your structure to the reader. Indeed, it is worth checking with your supervisor because some universities discourage the use of headings and subheadings, while other assignments require a clear structure and headings. You should include 'signposting' statements at key points to help the reader understand what has been discussed and what you are moving on to; for example, 'Having defined partnership working, the next step is to discuss how each agency has a different role'. These are statements that indicate a transition between sections by reminding the reader of what has already been discussed and indicating what will be discussed next.

Literature reviews in empirical studies

If you are collecting your own data, your literature review needs to make an argument for your proposed research. In particular, it needs to address directly your research question and how you intend to respond to it. Aveyard (2010) makes the useful suggestion to insert your research question in the header and footer section of your document to ensure that you maintain your focus. Do not be tempted to extend out to issues that are interesting but outside your research question. Rather than a wide-ranging discussion of all the topics that could be relevant to your study, you should aim to produce a focused piece of work that makes the argument for your proposed study. This will often include gaps in the previous literature or methodological innovations that you would like to introduce.

Designing your research study will require you to make active choices and you need to show how these decisions were informed by your literature review. So, as well as the literature on your topic, you need to discuss the methodological literature. Whether this is included in your literature review or your methodology section will depend upon your individual research project and the approach of your university, so it is advisable to check this out with your supervisor.

A note on terminology

There are a number of common confusions in terminology that relate to how you use referencing in your literature review:

- Reference list versus bibliography: a common confusion is between a reference list and a bibliography; these are often used as if they are interchangeable terms. A reference list includes only those texts that you have cited in the main body of your literature. A bibliography includes all the texts that you have read whilst preparing your literature review, whether or not you have cited them. You will always need to provide a reference list, but you are not always required to provide a bibliography. Indeed, if your university uses the standard Harvard system (i.e. author name and date in text), a bibliography is not normally required.

- Citation versus references: another potential source of confusion is between a citation and a reference. The term 'citation' refers to the text within the main body of your literature review that informs the reader of which texts you are drawing upon (e.g. Begum, 2005, page 25). Strictly speaking, references refer to the systematic list of texts at the end of your literature review that includes all of the texts that you have cited, but it is often used informally as synonymous with a citation.
- Footnotes versus endnotes: footnotes and endnotes are usually in the form of numbered entries embedded in the main part of the text which direct the reader to a separate note at the foot of the page (footnotes) or a separate list at the end of the document (endnotes). They have traditionally been used for additional material, such as comments, thoughts and anecdotes that were not considered important enough to include in the main body of the text.

Using reference management software

There are a number of software packages available to help you manage your references. Current examples include Endnote, Mendeley, RefWorks, Papers and CiteULike. These are constantly developing and web-based versions have been developed using cloud technology that enables you to use the software from any computer.

Reference management software generally works as a database, collecting together the references for all the material that you are using to write your literature review. They link with word-processing software such as Microsoft Word, enabling you to insert citations in the main body of your text and automatically generate a reference list at the end of your text. This reduces the risk of one of the most frequent problems with academic coursework, namely, inaccurate reference lists. It is common for lecturers to mark work that has a reference list that does not include all of the material cited but instead includes additional material that the student intended to use but never got round to including.

Another advantage of reference management software is that some of the texts are likely to be used in other academic work so the material can be reused. Ideally, students should learn to use reference management software at the beginning of their studies to gain maximum benefit, but final-year students can get immediate benefits and hopefully will return for further study.

Some packages offer additional features. For example, Mendeley enables the user to store articles in a similar way to the music management software iTunes. When articles are imported in PDF format, the software automatically recognises key information (journal title, year, author, title and so on) and the article can be tagged and arranged into bibliographies or 'playlists' for different projects. Articles can be shared with other users, who can be invited to view specific material or the whole database of articles. When choosing reference management software, it is worth checking out these additional features.

Some common challenges when writing a literature review

There are a number of challenges that students can experience whilst completing their literature reviews.

How do I decide what to include and what to leave out?

One of the most common problems with literature reviews is that students try to use every piece of material that they have read. This is at least partly because considerable work has gone into identifying and reading the material and the student wants the marker to know this. Although it can be disheartening to leave out material that you have worked hard on, it is almost essential to do this if you want to write a good literature review. The marker will want you to demonstrate that you are developing the ability to construct an argument, which requires you to include only material that is directly relevant to the points that you are making.

How far should I go back?

How far you go back depends entirely upon your research focus; for example, including classic studies could be highly relevant for some research projects. You can include a time limit on how far you go back, but you need to provide a justification for this; sometimes modules will specify a time limit such as within the last ten years. Whichever approach you take, you are expected to have a good grasp of current developments. If you have no material from the last ten years, it may appear that you have not developed your literature-searching skills sufficiently. It is possible that there really is no literature from the last decade, but you need to explain this and what measures you have taken to find it.

What if I search for literature relating to my topic and there is not a great deal out there?

It is always helpful to be explicit in your dissertation about how you conducted your literature search. For example, 'I used the Medline, Cochrane and Applied Social Sciences Index Abstracts (ASSIA) databases using the following search terms: x, y, z.' This makes the process transparent and enables the reader to see exactly what you did. This is particularly important if the literature that you identify is rather limited, because it helps convince the reader that you have undertaken a concerted and systematic attempt to identify relevant material. If your literature is extremely sparse, you need to consider whether you've chosen a suitable topic for your project, because it can be difficult to write your literature review and for you to discuss the significance of your findings without responding to a body of literature, and it can be complex and confusing using related but not directly relevant literature to construct an argument.

What if my original literature review does not cover (or match) all of the issues that came out in the data?

If your literature review forms part of an empirical research study, you may find that you need to revise your literature review because your data have highlighted issues that were not in your original literature review. This is quite common in qualitative studies, where your research is more exploratory. Occasionally there can be a serious mismatch between the original literature review and the issues identified in the data analysis which requires a significant reworking of the literature review. The most common reason for this is that the questions used at data collection stage (e.g. interview or focus group questions) were not clearly linked into the literature review so they cover different topics. Once the data are analysed, the issues raised need to be the focus of a revised literature review. The simplest remedy is to ensure that your data collection questions are informed by and relate to the issues identified in your literature review. For most research projects, the revisions are relatively minor but do ensure that you allow yourself sufficient time at the writing-up stage.

Writing up your documentary analysis

This builds upon Chapter 2, where we started exploring documentary analysis as a research method. It was emphasised that a documentary analysis is quite different from a literature review because it is a form of primary research in its own right. This distinction was discussed and the process of undertaking a documentary analysis was outlined, using a case study to illustrate the stages. The criteria for judging documents when selecting your sample were discussed and guidelines for sampling were provided.

Using content analysis in documentary analysis

Content analysis is one of the most common analytical designs employed in documentary analysis. It is a popular choice at least partly because it provides a relatively straightforward way of making sense of textual data by converting them into a quantifiable form. However, there are a range of different approaches within the qualitative tradition (Miles and Huberman, 1994). These include approaches such as clinical data mining (Epstein, 2010), discourse analysis (Potter and Wetherell, 1987; Parker, 1992), narrative analysis (Riessman, 1993, 2007; Andrews et al., 2008) and semiotics (Barthes, 1972; Saussure, 1983). Content analysis and documentary analysis are included in this chapter as their basic units of analysis are words in the form of text. Documents are thus similar to interview transcripts but content analysis is a quantitative process used to analyse them which can also be used on interview transcripts, but with completely different results compared to the qualitative processes described above.

What is content analysis?

An established definition is that content analysis is *a research technique for the objective, systematic and quantitative description of the manifest content of communication* (Berelson, 1952, page 18). As the quotation suggests, content analysis uses objective and systematic counting and recording procedures to produce quantitative data about the manifest (i.e. visible) content of communication. It is most commonly used in the analysis of mass communication, but it is a versatile research method (Bryman, 2012).

One of the key choices that researchers must make in content analysis is the extent to which manifest and latent coding are used. *Manifest coding* refers to analysing the visible, explicit content of a text, a relatively straightforward process of counting the relative frequency of particular terms. However, it presupposes that different texts use the same or similar terms. *Latent coding* refers to analysing the implicit content of a text and it involves a degree of interpretation to uncover the meanings that lie beneath the words in the text.

We will return to the case study of Sarah, who is interested in how the media portray people with mental health problems. (Sarah was introduced in Chapter 2 and we discussed her work earlier in this chapter.) You heard about the first two stages of a documentary analysis: choosing a research question and deciding which documents to include in the sample. Sarah decided that she wanted to focus upon women with a diagnosis of schizophrenia and to study how they were portrayed by the media. She chose to analyse newspaper reports through an electronic database, selecting a randomised 10% sample of the 600 newspaper reports involving people diagnosed with schizophrenia in 2013. Now she must make a choice about whether she will use manifest or latent coding.

Case study: Choosing coding for analysis

One of the issues that she wishes to investigate is whether newspapers use discriminatory language when reporting news stories about people diagnosed with schizophrenia. If she wishes to use manifest coding, she would develop a list of specific discriminatory terms that she would look for. If she wishes to use latent coding, she would take into account implied meanings that would suggest that the individual is being viewed negatively even if the article was not explicitly discriminatory.

If Sarah chooses manifest coding, she risks missing news stories where discrimination is present but not explicit. If she chooses latent coding, she risks misinterpreting subtle meanings that are implied but not explicit. Like many research decisions, there is no 'right' answer; she must simply make a decision and give her rationale for it.

Advantages and disadvantages of content analysis

Content analysis has a number of strengths and weaknesses. Content analysis is able to quantify the content of texts in a transparent and clear way (Denscombe, 2007; Bryman, 2012). The procedures are relatively objective and exhibit reliability because they can be replicated by others. It is a flexible method, particularly suited to longitudinal studies, which study phenomena over time (see Clements and Foster (2008) for a good example). It can reveal hidden aspects of what is being communicated because researchers can code for aspects that are not included in the text (e.g. analysing luxury car adverts for images of people from minority ethnic communities).

Content analysis has been criticised for being a crude instrument because of its tendency to remove text from its context, which risks losing some of its complex and subtle meanings; certainly there will not be the depth and complexity in the data analysis and findings compared to using a qualitative technique such as thematic analysis. As a result, it is regarded as being most appropriate when what you are studying is relatively straightforward, clear and observable (Denscombe, 2007). The use of latent coding provides more flexibility and allows data to be viewed in its context, but is controversial because it introduces a level of interpretation. One way in which this can be addressed is by establishing interrater reliability through having multiple coders and checking whether different coders identify the same meanings. As with other forms of quantitative research, content analysis can describe phenomena and identify trends but we can usually only speculate about the reasons. A final criticism is the tendency to focus on what is measurable rather than what is theoretically significant. This is captured by a quotation that Einstein is reputed to have kept on his office wall:

> *Not everything that can be counted counts, and not everything that counts can be counted.*

Collecting and analysing data in a documentary analysis

A key decision in documentary analysis is the basic unit of analysis; that is, the amount of text to be using for coding, such as a single word, phrase, sentence or a whole article (Neuman, 2006). In our case study, Sarah has decided to use a whole newspaper article as her research unit.

Second, a codebook and a recording sheet are required. A codebook is a set of instructions for coders that explains how documents are going to be coded. This includes guidance as to what is included under each dimension and what coders should take into account when deciding how to allocate a particular code. The aim of the codebook is to ensure that all documents are coded consistently and in a way that can be replicated by others. Sarah's codebook would look like the one shown in Figure 9.1. (In real life, the study would look at a larger range of variables but it has been simplified to demonstrate the process.)

When coding data, it is generally accepted (Sarantakos, 2005; Neuman, 2006) that there are four dimensions to consider: frequency, direction, prominence and intensity. Not all of the dimensions may be relevant and researchers may measure from one of these to all four dimensions (Neuman, 2006).

1. Frequency: was the required unit of research present? For the case study, this would mean deciding whether schizophrenia was mentioned in the news article.
2. Direction: was it positive, negative or neutral? This involves rating the content of the message along a scale. For the case study, this would mean whether the article presented the person diagnosed with schizophrenia in a positive, negative or neutral way.
3. Prominence: what prominence was given in the document? For Sarah's project, was the news story the front-page headline or was it on page 14?
4. Intensity: how powerful was the message? This measures the extent to which the unit of research is stressed. For Sarah, this would be the extent to which the person's mental health problem was stressed in the article.

Codebook

Case ID: case identification number for article, numbered sequentially

Gender of person with a diagnosis of schizophrenia in the news story

Please insert one of the following codes:
1 = female
2 = male
0 = not specified

Tabloid or broadsheet newspaper

Please insert one of the following codes:
1 = broadsheet
2 = tabloid

Name of publication

Glasgow category, i.e. categories developed by the Glasgow Media Group (1996)
1 = Violence to others
2 = Harm to self
3 = Prescriptive/advice
4 = Criticism of accepted definitions of mental illness
5 = 'Comic' images
6 = Other

Stigmatising language
0 = no stigmatising language
1 = stigmatising language

Prominence (location in publication)
1 = front page
2 = pages 2 or 3
3 = other page

Intensity (extent to which person's mental health problem was stressed)
1 = Low
2 = Medium
3 = High

Figure 9.1: Codebook

The next stage is to design a recording sheet in order to document the results of coding. Once a coding manual has been designed, analysis can begin by taking the first document and starting to code it; that is, identifying and classifying the aspects of the document that have been identified and writing this down on the recording sheet. In the case study, Sarah's recording sheet would look like the one shown in Figure 9.2. (This has been simplified to illustrate the process and a real-life study would look at a wider range of variables.)

A spreadsheet package such as Excel is often used to develop a coding schedule which can record and analyse data and can be exported into statistical software packages such as SPSS. Quantitative data are normally presented in the form of tables and graphs, which are discussed in detail in Chapter 7.

Case ID	Gender	Tabloid or broadsheet	Publication	Glasgow category	Stigmatising language	Prominence	Intensity
1	2	1	Times	1	1	1	2
2	1	2	Mail	2	0	3	3
3	2	2	Mail	1	1	2	3
4	2	1	Independent	1	1	1	1
5	1	1	Guardian	4	1	1	2
6	2	2	Mail	1	1	1	2

Figure 9.2: Recording sheet

Chapter summary

In this chapter, we looked at how to write up a literature review and how to analyse and write a documentary analysis. In the first part, we examined the different purposes of a literature review, both as a stand-alone piece of work and as part of an empirical research project. We looked at different ways of structuring your literature review and explored how reference management software can be helpful.

There were a number of key messages. Ensure that you provide a clear account of how you undertook your literature search so that the reader knows that your search was systematic and rigorous. It is important that you signpost your literature review at each stage, so readers know what to expect and what you have already covered.

In the second part of this chapter, we examined how you can analyse and write up your documentary analysis. We focused on content analysis as a relatively rigorous and accessible approach and discussed the strengths and weaknesses of this approach.

Activity answer

9.1: Critical thinking (page 156)

As a first draft, Sarah's original statement is too much like a list of the available literature rather than a critical appraisal of it. Studies are described separately, with no attempt to create an overall narrative. An alternative paragraph could be:

> *The prevalence of discriminatory language varies in different forms of media (Begum, 2001; Jones, 2005; Bhutto, 2008). In one study of one month of UK news coverage on ten television channels and all UK national newspapers, Bhutto (2008) found that newspapers were 72% more likely to use discriminatory language. In a previous study, Begum (2001) used a similar design over a one-week period using all UK national tabloid newspapers and found that tabloid newspapers were almost four times as likely to use discriminatory language in news items about women with mental health problems. Although the*

two studies used different time periods, Bhutto (2008) argues that the significant difference in results is primarily due to her including all national newspapers rather than just tabloids.

If this issue was central to Sarah's research question, she would discuss it in more detail and would probably write a paragraph for each study and discuss methodological issues in depth.

Further reading

Literature reviews

Aveyard, H (2010) *Doing a Literature Review in Health and Social Care*, 2nd edition. Berkshire: Open University Press.
A useful and rigorous account of conducting a literature review.

Hart, C (1998) *Doing a Literature Review: Releasing the Social Science Research Imagination.* London: Sage.
A classic text on compiling your literature review that gives detailed guidance on structure and evaluating arguments.

Ridley, D (2012) *The Literature Review: A Step-by-Step Guide for Students,* 2nd edition. London: Sage.
A useful and readable account.

Documentary analysis

Atkinson, P and Coffey, A (2004) Analysing documentary realities, in D Silverman (ed.) *Qualitative Research: Theory, Method and Practice,* 2nd edition. London: Sage.
Interesting and useful discussion about documentary analysis from a qualitative perspective.

Epstein, I (2010) *Clinical Data-Mining: Integrating Practice and Research.* Oxford: Oxford University Press.
An excellent and interesting account of a new approach to documentary analysis, including practical examples of previous clinical data-mining studies. An insightful and entertaining read, likely to become a classic.

Prior, L (2003) *Using Documents in Social Research.* London: Sage.
Detailed account of documentary analysis from a qualitative perspective. Interesting discussion of a philosophical basis for documentary analysis.

Scott, J (1990) *A Matter of Record: Documentary Sources in Social Research.* Cambridge: Polity Press.
A classic text in documentary analysis, concentrating mainly on historical documents.

Useful websites

http://www.casp-uk.net
The Critical Appraisal Skills Programme (CASP) supports an evidence-based approach in health and social care and has developed a number of tools to help with the process of critically appraising articles. The website contains evaluation tools for a range of approaches, including systematic reviews, randomised controlled trials, qualitative research, economic evaluation studies and diagnostic test studies.

www.proquest.com
ProQuest is a national electronic database of newspaper articles from a range of national tabloid and broadsheet newspapers. Normally available through your university library webpage.

Chapter 10
Writing your research proposal and dissertation

Chapter aims

After reading this chapter, you should be able to:

- feel confident about writing up your dissertation;
- feel confident about writing a proposal;
- understand the different skills needed for presenting quantitative and qualitative research.

Introduction

In this chapter we will do two things: we will introduce you to some basic skills in writing (relating these to writing a dissertation), and we will give you some tips about how to write a research proposal. As most of this book has been written from the perspective of planning a project, including tips on how to write up a finished project may seem odd, but these points are relevant to anyone writing a large and extensive piece of work. Indeed, in some institutions an extended study such as a research proposal and literature review is considered to be a form of dissertation, even though no data have been collected.

We will look first at skills relevant to writing a dissertation, including some general advice about writing *per se*, before finishing off with looking at specific issues relating to a proposal. The differences between presenting quantitative and qualitative research will be outlined.

Writing a dissertation

A dissertation or research proposal and literature review is likely to be the longest piece of independent work that you will submit for your course, so compliance with the university's requirements is essential.

The process of writing

Writing up your research dissertation can be both exciting and daunting because it is unlike your previous coursework in three ways. First, it has a structure and terminology that are unlike the standard essay format. Second, it is likely to be a long piece of work, longer than an essay and usually completed with some element of self-directed study over a longer time period than normal. Third, it is likely that you will have some form of one-to-one tutorial support from a lecturer; this is often called supervision.

The writing process itself can be a source of anxiety. Becker describes running a seminar on writing skills and found that students identified two main fears:

> *They were afraid that they would not be able to organise their thoughts, that writing would be a big confused chaos that would drive them mad. They spoke feelingly about a second fear, that what they wrote would be 'wrong' and that (unspecified) people would laugh at them.*
> (Becker, 2007, page 4)

Becker (2007) found that students adopted a number of coping mechanisms to manage their anxiety. For example, using particular pens or paper, sharpening pencils or cleaning the house (he found a gender divide on the latter!).

Activity 10.1 — *Reflection*

Can you relate to these fears? Are there different concerns and anxieties you have about writing?

As this activity is for your own reflection, there is no outline answer given.

You may have been able to see yourself in Becker's comments. Or there may be other anxieties and concerns that you were able to identify. The important point is not to let yourself be paralysed by your anxieties.

One common barrier is the belief that you must read everything that is written on your topic and work out your ideas before you put them down. The danger is that writing will be continually postponed while you read and think some more. Start writing as soon as you can because the writing process helps to identify your thoughts. Becker expresses it well:

> *Writing a dissertation starts with writing, not with preparing to write . . . And feeling unready is no excuse at all. In scholarship, one is never ready, since there is always something else that one can sensibly read. All scholarship, strictly speaking, is at first written by the unprepared, or at least by the under-prepared . . . Since you are never ready to write, you start writing before you are ready.*
> (Becker, 1986, page 88)

Delamont et al. (2004) offer two golden rules for writing your dissertation:

1. Write early and write often: the more you write, the easier it gets and it becomes a habit. The later you leave it to start writing, the more difficult it can become. Work out the times that you are most productive and try to develop a routine of writing something every day.

2. Don't get it right, get it written: drafting is an essential stage in working out what you want to say. In previous smaller essays on single topics, it may have been possible to hold everything in your head while you plan. With a dissertation, you have simply too much material, and often a series of related topics that you progressively develop, so drafting is an essential part of the process of working out what you want to say. As you write, you are likely to see some of the tensions, contradictions and inconsistencies in your argument (Delamont et al., 2004, page 121).

Free writing, in which you write down whatever comes into your head without censoring or editing, can help you to establish what you want to say without being paralysed by choices (Becker, 2007). It also helps you realise that you can write your ideas down without fear, and that the only draft that counts is the final draft.

Activity 10.2　　　　　　　　　　　　　　　　　　　　　*Reflection*

Write for 5–10 minutes about your thoughts and feelings concerning writing up your dissertation and what barriers you envisage. If you run out of things to say, repeat your last word continuously until further words come to you.

As this activity is for your own reflection, there is no outline answer given.

This is a useful exercise for two reasons. First, you experience the process of free writing and discover how liberating and frightening it can be to write whatever comes into your head. It can be a powerful lesson in how we often do not know what we think about a subject until we see what we have written down on the page. Second, the content of what you have written helps you to understand the potential barriers to you completing your dissertation. These barriers can be physical; for example, finding and protecting the time given the other demands of the course and your personal and work life. They can also be psychological, such as the fear that you will not be able to produce academic work of the standard required. This fear is particularly common and can partly explain why dissertations are often delayed more than other pieces of coursework (although other reasons, such as delays in getting ethical approval or access to participants, are at least as important). Identifying these barriers will help you plan to overcome them. One common way of planning your writing is to use a SWOT analysis (strengths, weaknesses, opportunities and threats; this is sometimes called a SCOT analysis, with C standing for challenges, but the principle is the same). If you are engaged in writing a dissertation, literature review and/or proposal, right at the very beginning sit down and spend a couple of hours writing a SWOT analysis. Include some concrete objectives with each element, giving them a timeframe as you work towards the final submission date. You might want to think about your skills in relation to the following areas:

- literature searching;
- critiquing research reports;
- concepts of evidence-based practice and clinical effectiveness;

- qualitative research concepts and methods;
- quantitative research concepts and methods;
- writing a research proposal;
- personal study skills and time management;
- use of information technologies.

Structuring your dissertation or proposal

Your university will provide you with specific guidelines for how to structure your dissertation, research proposal or project, and these will be in the relevant module handbook or study guide. Make sure that you adhere to them to the letter! This is particularly true if your university has developed a structure that is specific to that module or programme. However, most universities use a traditional dissertation format and provide less detailed guidance, so this chapter will be important for helping you know how to structure your work.

The traditional dissertation layout has the format given below. A proposal will not have a findings section, but instead may include sections on clinical relevance, dissemination and risks to the project:

1. Title page: check your university's rules about the exact format.
2. Table of contents: this provides a clear guide to where readers can find particular sections.
3. Abstract: this provides a summary of your research, including a brief account of your research design and findings. In a proposal there will not be any findings.
4. Introduction: this should introduce your research question and explain why it is important. It should outline your approach and clarify the structure of the dissertation.
5. Literature review: this is a coherent and critical account of the literature that provides an overall argument based upon your reading of the literature.
6. Methodology: this explains in clear and specific terms how you conducted your research. It includes an overview of what you did, why you made your choices and how you addressed ethical issues. For proposals these will be in the future tense ('I plan to use an action research methodology').
7. Findings and discussion: in quantitative dissertations, the presentation of findings is usually separated from the discussion section, while they are combined for qualitative research.
8. Conclusion: the conclusion should summarise your research and its major components together with a summary of the principal findings and how they relate to the literature. The conclusion could include recommendations for policy and practice and for future research, listing possible areas of inquiry.
9. References: these should be set out in the appropriate format for your university.
10. Appendices: these include additional background information, such as your interview schedule or questionnaire and sample information sheets given to participants.

Writing your abstract

Although your abstract appears first, it is written last. Abstracts are commonly 250–350 words and the aim is to condense your research project into a short summary. Your abstract contains the basic message of your research and should include your research question or topic, methodology, findings and their significance for the field.

Look at the journal articles that you have read for your literature review. Each contains an abstract that is carefully crafted because the authors know that most readers will search the literature using bibliographic databases containing abstracts only. If the abstract is badly written and unclear, few readers will take the time to read the whole article. Use them as examples to inform your writing. Some journals (like the *Journal of Advanced Nursing* and the *Journal of Clinical Nursing*) also have a summary section which asks authors to indicate what is already known and what this piece adds. This might be useful as part of the abstract, as might the inclusion of three or four key words.

Writing your introduction

This should introduce your research question and explain why it is important. Stating that it is a long-standing interest for you is not enough on its own, although this could be part of a rationale for undertaking the study; indeed, frequently students will be asked to choose an area from their practice that they want to investigate further. This gives it a personal, clinical focus that is highly valuable in nursing.

As a general guide, your introduction should start with your main aims and provide a short summary of the background context of your study. Frequently there is a policy context that should be acknowledged in the introduction, whereas the literature review section will review a body of research literature, systematic reviews and guidelines (if there are any). The introduction should be clear about the main problem or issues to be investigated and present your overall approach. Finally, you should provide a short description of the structure of your dissertation (Walliman, 2006).

You do not have to start writing by working on the introduction. Indeed, there are good arguments for writing your introduction last, because it is at that stage that you will have a good idea of what you are going to say. It is not uncommon to read dissertation introductions that state that a particular topic will be discussed, then find that the main body of the dissertation is about a different topic. This is usually because the writer has developed his or her thinking and discovered that the research is really about the second topic rather than the first topic. This is a healthy part of the research process, but you need to ensure that you redraft your introduction to reflect this.

Writing your literature review

Chapter 9 covers this in detail but, to recap, a popular approach is the chronological structure, which begins with the early development of the field and progresses through to the most recent developments. For example, Patrick is interested in the barriers to fathers being involved in parenting assessments. His literature review discusses previous writing on the involvement of fathers where there are child welfare concerns. A chronological structure examines how the topic has been discussed during different time periods.

Alternatively, Patrick could adopt a thematic approach that focuses on particular issues identified in the literature, such as media representations of fatherhood or the growing awareness of domestic violence. This could have a funnel structure, looking at the wider context of policy and public perceptions of fathers and progressively narrowing down to the involvement of fathers in parenting assessments. Either structure is acceptable and good dissertations will give a clear rationale for the structure selected.

Some universities might expect you to conduct a systematic review of the literature. In that case you will need to give search terms, databases and numbers of hits, and your inclusion and exclusion criteria. It may be possible to discuss findings from this approach chronologically, but a thematic structure would be more impressive, so that you can group papers by their underlying theme. These can be summarised in an appendix to indicate how thoroughly you have reviewed the literature, as shown in Table 10.1.

Full reference	Study aims and design	Methods of data collection and analysis	Results	Comments
Lock CA, Kaner E, Heather N, Doughty J, Crawshaw A, McNamee P, Purdy S & Pearson P (2006) Effectiveness of nurse-led brief alcohol intervention: a cluster randomized controlled trial. *Journal of Advanced Nursing* 54 (4): 426–439	A pragmatic cluster randomised controlled trial was carried out to evaluate the effects of a brief intervention compared with standard advice (the control group)	Excessive consumption was identified opportunistically via the Alcohol Use Disorders Identification Test. After baseline assessment, patients received either a 5–10-minutes brief intervention using the 'Drink Less' protocol or standard advice (control condition). Follow-up occurred at 6 and 12 months postintervention	There were no statistically significant differences between intervention and control patients at follow-up	
And so on!				

Table 10.1: How to present a brief summary of papers as an appendix

Rather than taking things at face value, a good literature review will address the contradictions and omissions in previous writing. Remember that what scores highly (and will probably be a module requirement in the last year of an undergraduate programme or in postgraduate studies) is a critical analysis and synthesis of the literature. So, what are your papers indicating as a body of literature? Are there key themes or issues to be identified? Are there strengths and weaknesses in their methodologies? What is the impact for your study of the methodological approach taken in the papers? (If you find only small-scale qualitative studies, is it time for a large-scale quantitative design, for example?)

Avoid phrases such as 'research tells us' unless you are prepared to state exactly which research studies you are referring to and provide some form of critical analysis of them. Your marker is unlikely to let vague references to unspecified research go unchallenged at this stage in your studies.

Writing your methodology section

Journalists are taught that the first sentence of a newspaper article should answer the following questions: who, what, when, where, why and sometimes how (Leki, 1998, page 25). While academic readers are likely to be more forgiving, these questions are useful to guide your methodology section. Your methodology section should usually address the following areas:

- Overall research approach and methods: what is/was your overall approach (qualitative or quantitative)? This is often referred to as your choice of paradigm, and can also be termed choice of methodology (as distinct from your methods). What research methods will you/did you use to collect your data (interviews, questionnaires, focus groups)? Why did you choose this approach and research method compared to alternative approaches?
- Sampling: who will/did you have as participants? What is/was the size and composition of your sample? How will/did you select and contact them? Where will/did you go to get access to them?
- Analysis: how will/did you analyse your data? Why will/did you choose that particular approach?
- Ethical issues: how will/did you address ethical issues, such as gaining access to participants or other sources of data, informed consent, confidentiality, anonymising data and ethical data management?
- Limitations: what are the limitations of your research? This discussion can begin here and be developed further in the discussion of your findings.

Presenting and discussing your qualitative data

Obviously if you have not collected data, you won't be doing this, but there are some points here that might inform your thinking about presenting qualitative data. In qualitative dissertations, the presentation of findings is in prose form and lends itself to being discussed immediately. Consequently, findings and discussion are usually combined into one section.

In Chapter 5, thematic analysis was outlined as a good model for analysing most forms of qualitative data. The six-stage model developed by Braun and Clarke (2006) was outlined and the first five stages were described in detail. Our focus in this chapter is on the final stage, writing up and presenting your analysis.

The final stage begins when you have established and refined your themes. Your task in writing up your analysis is to tell the complicated story of your data in a way which convinces the reader of the merit and validity of your analysis (Braun and Clarke, 2006, page 93). Your aim is to provide a concise and coherent narrative that contains sufficient quotes that demonstrate your themes without becoming repetitive. Do not present your quotes without explanation and expect readers to make the connections themselves. Just as you would make an argument and provide a quote from a book or article as evidence to strengthen your argument, use the quotes from your participants in a similar way. Choose particularly vivid and concise quotes that demonstrate your point as closely as possible. Better to have one or perhaps two crisp quotes than include three or four more general quotes. Your quotes need to illustrate a narrative that presents an argument about how the data respond to your research question.

Your findings should be organised according to the themes identified in your analysis rather than just using your interview or focus group questions as a structure. If you just summarise what participants said in response to question one, two and so on, this presents an impression that you have merely described your data rather than analysed them. Avoid using statistics to present your findings when you have small sample sizes. Stating '80% of participants' sounds more dramatic than 'four out of five participants' but your reader is aware of your sample size and is unlikely to be convinced.

The key ethical issue in your findings section is protecting the confidentiality of your participants. The highest risk is often when you use a quote and identify a participant by a characteristic, such as the person's role, gender, ethnicity or sexual orientation. If the group that the participant belongs to is small, there is a high risk that other participants or other interested parties would be able to identify him or her. Consequently, avoid identifying a participant in this way; it rarely detracts significantly from your analysis. If you feel that you must, you may need to show your final draft to the participant to obtain his or her permission.

Presenting and discussing your quantitative data

We have looked at descriptive and inferential statistics in Chapter 7, so what follows are some general points about presenting quantitative data. In quantitative research, the presentation of findings is in table and graph form so it is conventional to split findings and discussion into two separate headings. A common practice is to include your raw data as an appendix at the back and draw upon the key data in the main body of your dissertation to illustrate your argument. Charts and tables should be in the body of the text, not as an appendix, otherwise it is difficult for readers to follow your argument.

Make your presentation of data attractive and clear. Always give a chart a title and make sure it is clear what it represents. Mark the axes to show scale and include legends to indicate figures or percentages. For a detailed discussion of the presentation of quantitative data, see Dunleavy (2003).

Although the general principles of presenting quantitative data are straightforward, it can take time to get it right. Indeed, Delamont et al. (2004) argue that you should 'expect to suffer' about the presentation of statistics. Although this may be pessimistic, do allow yourself sufficient time. It is likely that you'll run various tests over and over again as you develop understanding of the possibilities of your computer program and your thinking develops about the study itself.

In quantitative research, a separate discussion section enables you to examine the significance of your findings. This can be compared to other studies or to theories in your field. The discussion of your findings enables you to revisit your original research question and explore what you have learnt.

Avoid over-generalising your findings. What you may find in one setting in one area at one point in time can rarely be generalised to all populations at all points in time and it is important to be clear about this in your findings section. Silverman captures this eloquently:

> *It always helps to make limited claims about your own research. Grandiose claims about originality, scope or applicability to social problems are all hostages to fortune. Be careful in how you specify the claims of your approach. Show that you understand that it constitutes one way of 'slicing the cake' and that other approaches, using other forms of data, may not be directly competitive.*
> (Silverman, 2013, page 49)

In research, it is always wise to be realistic about what you can claim based upon your evidence and better to understate rather than overstate your findings.

For both forms of data analysis, in your discussion make sure that you are clear about how your findings answer your research questions, and make sure that you link and discuss how your study sits in relation to the body of literature. This can be done by noting how your findings equate with other work in the field and may involve you revisiting some of the literature you used to justify the study in the literature review section. It may also require you to draw on extra references to literature that you have not already discussed.

Writing your conclusion

The conclusion should summarise your research and its major components together with a summary of the principal findings and how it relates to the literature. You should not introduce new material at this stage but should summarise complex arguments you have given in the discussion. Your conclusion could discuss lessons learnt from the process of research as well as the findings. Your conclusion could include recommendations for education, policy and practice in your research area. It could also include recommendations for future research, listing possible areas of inquiry or research designs. Try to be specific rather than simply stating that 'further research should be done'.

Some general points
Should I use 'I' in my dissertation?

Traditionally, students were encouraged to use the passive voice; for example, 'the research interviews were conducted with six participants', rather than the active voice, 'I conducted interviews with six participants'. Students were particularly instructed to avoid using 'I' because it appeared too informal and not compatible with the 'scientific' tone expected. Within quantitative research using a positivist approach, this convention is usually still observed, though the active voice is more acceptable than using 'I'. In qualitative research, the active voice is encouraged and 'I' is used more frequently, because reflexivity is actively encouraged.

Your choice should be guided by whether your research is quantitative or qualitative and by the expectations of your university and supervisor. If you do choose to use 'I', use it sparingly. Avoid overuse; for example, 'I think that I found that I was approaching my topic because I feel I had previously viewed my beliefs . . . '. Use 'I' when it genuinely adds something to what you are saying.

Structuring your dissertation

This is not just about headings. A good dissertation includes clear signposting. Since you are taking your reader on a journey, it is important to provide clear statements about where you are going and where you have been. At the end of each section, recap and tell the reader what you will be discussing next.

The function of sentences and paragraphs

A sentence is used to express a single idea. If a sentence expresses two or more ideas, you are probably making it work too hard. Try splitting it into two sentences for greater clarity.

A paragraph consists of several sentences grouped together to express a set of related ideas. Consequently, one-sentence paragraphs are to be avoided.

Knowing what to leave out

Do not feel that you have to use every piece of material that you have gathered through the research process. The marker will want you to show you can construct an argument and use material selectively. This requires you to leave out material that is not relevant, which is much better than trying to 'shoehorn' extraneous material into your dissertation because you have expended considerable effort in obtaining it. A good researcher knows that the quality of research is as much about what is left out as what is included.

Referencing and proofreading your work

Referencing in your dissertation is no different to an essay or another piece of academic work. Most UK universities have adopted the Harvard referencing system and have produced help sheets to provide guidance. Check with your university website or library. Even if you know the Harvard system well, it is worthwhile checking because there are minor differences between universities about how they have interpreted the Harvard system. Many students feel that this is relatively unimportant, but good referencing does impress markers so it is well worth learning how to reference accurately.

One of the most common mistakes is for your references to omit texts that you have cited and to include texts that you have not cited. This is usually because you have included your references as you have worked on your drafts, but not checked them at the end. So, as you have reworked your material, you have cut out material but left the original references in. Conversely, you have included material that cites texts that you have not yet put in your references. This mismatch between dissertation and references is surprisingly common, even with otherwise diligent students. To check you have the right references in it, it is useful to go through each page, making sure that those that are there are listed in the reference section.

As you write, ensure that you save your work frequently and keep back-up copies. As a general rule, keep a back-up copy on one or more removable drives and email yourself a copy regularly. This ensures that, even if your computer and removable drives were destroyed, you would still have a copy of your work.

Finally, careful proofreading is always worthwhile because it makes it easier for readers to understand what you are saying. Try to complete your dissertation before the deadline. This enables you to sleep on it and reread your dissertation with fresh eyes. Ideally, enlist another person because he or she is more likely to identify mistakes or confusions that you may miss.

If you have checked your spelling and grammar, markers are more likely to notice what you have to say, rather than being distracted by poor presentation and typing mistakes. Coco Chanel reputedly said: *Dress shabbily and they remember the dress; dress impeccably and they remember the woman.* The same is true of writing.

Disseminating and publishing your work

Completing your dissertation is a significant achievement. Having met the requirements of your degree, it may be tempting just to put it proudly on your bookshelf. However, it is worth considering how to disseminate your research to a wider audience. Managers, colleagues, service users and carers are all stakeholders who could benefit from hearing the results of your research. This can range from a presentation or short summary to writing for a professional or academic publication. If you are considering this, speak to your supervisor, who may be able to provide useful help and advice. It is unlikely that a student could get a piece published in a reputable academic journal without help, so an experienced academic with a good publication record in that type of journal should help you. Your supervisor might suggest that you try to publish if your work is good. In that case, the usual arrangement is that you would take first authorship and the supervisor second. If you enjoyed your research project, you may also want to discuss opportunities for further research with your supervisor, either independently or as a part of further study.

Having looked at writing skills which are relevant to any type of writing, we will now examine some tips specifically for proposal writing.

Proposal writing tips

Wong (2005) has a number of suggestions that relate specifically to proposal writing. He argues that students frequently do not understand how important a proposal is and how its quality influences one's chances of success: without knowing what you are doing in advance and having clearly defined your methodology and methods of data collection and analysis, you will be adrift without a compass when it comes to actually doing the work. A proposal should show that your research is worth doing and that you have the knowledge and skills to complete it successfully: apart from these practicalities, it is unethical for an institution to allow students to undertake research if they don't know how or why they are collecting data, or what they are going to do with it, as this exposes participants to unnecessary, unjustified or unwise procedures. Obviously, then, your proposal should contain all the elements involved in the research process, with enough material at the correct level for your programme of study so that readers and markers can assess why the study is needed, what you plan to do and how you plan to do it (Wong, 2005). This can be achieved by a thorough literature review and critical analysis, accurate and appropriate specification of the methodology and methods, addressing ethical considerations rather than just saying 'ethical approval will be obtained', and writing in a structure that addresses the assessment and/or institutional requirements. It should also be written in a coherent and engaging manner that has correct standards of English, grammar and punctuation, and has been effectively proofread. Another useful tip is to get someone with more experience to read it. This could be a researcher or, more likely for students, a supervisor or module lecturer. The title is also very important and should be informative, convey clearly what the proposal is about, reflect the overall methodological approach, and usually (although not necessarily) be a sentence with a question mark at the end. As always, the question drives the study design, not the other way around!

How different titles can convey entirely different methodological approaches in proposals

1. What are the differences in effectiveness between silver-coated urinary catheters and antibiotic-coated catheters?

Comment

This question is clearly asking whether there are differences between groups. The researchers want to know which type of product works best, so they would construct a null hypothesis that there are no differences between groups and seek to falsify (disprove) it. Methodologically, the way to assess this is to use an experimental design; thus the question drives the choice of study design, not the other way around. There would be a range of outcomes which could be measures, such as infection rates, rates of clogging/ blockage, cost-effectiveness and lengths of time of insertion.

2. What are patients' experiences of living with a long-term urinary catheter?

Comment

Here, there is no sense in which a hypothesis can be tested, as the question is asking for patients' experiences. A qualitative study design would be used in order to get a rich and indepth perspective of what it is like to live with a urinary catheter in the long term. Individual interviews could be used, with data transcribed and thematically analysed.

3. How satisfied are patients with the urology service?

Comment

This is a different issue from the two above as the researchers are trying to evaluate a service from the perspective of patients. This could be done using a questionnaire survey. It is neither an experimental design or an indepth qualitative approach, but could use an existing satisfaction measure, or a specially designed one, using a mix of Likert-scale questions with some free-text open-ended ones.

4. How effective are nurses' infection control techniques concerning insertion and care of urinary catheters? An observational study.

Comment

This question contains specific reference to the method to be used, which is observation. This makes it completely clear what the researchers are planning to do and leaves the reader in no doubt about what to expect from the proposal.

Timetable

Every proposal must include a timetable. This shows the timeframe to which you will be working. This is most important in any setting, but particularly so if you have to meet coursework deadlines. You will need to plan carefully, and plan on a weekly or monthly basis each step that you will take. Most proposals will have clear steps that mirror the research process, and you will need to allocate these times for starting and finishing. Figure 3.2 on page 56 shows how you can construct a simple timetable using a Microsoft Word table. A more sophisticated and impressive way of presenting your timetable is to use a Gantt chart. Figure 10.1 shows an example of a Gantt chart.

There are many different software packages freely available for doing this if you search the internet, and it can also be achieved using Microsoft Excel.

Resources

A proposal will also need some estimation of resources. If you were submitting your proposal for funding, this would need to be very accurate. Universities and NHS Trusts have teams of dedicated staff to do this, and you should ask them to do it for you if you are looking for funding in reality. Universities are now subject to something called Full Economic Costing (FEC) in research bids and this is a complicated area, so let the accountants get it right for you! In a students' proposal, it would be necessary only to estimate, not cost, the types of resources you might need, such as staff, computers, statistician time, room rental, travel and subsistence costs, and so on.

Figure 10.1: Gantt chart for project planning. Adapted from an original diagram by Garry L Booker (8 October 2007)

Benefits and risks

Some proposal structures will ask you to discuss the benefits of your research, and this can be listed for the local NHS services, nationally and possibly even internationally (although you may need to wait until you are a professor before your work has impact internationally). You may also be asked to list risks in terms of the research to patients, but also in terms of the research not being completed: what happens if you can't recruit? Do you have a plan B?

Dissemination

Finally, it is time for you to think about the best way to publicise your work. Can it be published as a report, or as an article or chapter in a larger academic publication? Could you present your findings at a conference or write it up for a project website? The opportunities are wide-ranging.

Chapter summary

In this chapter, the key messages are to start writing early and to use the writing process to help you work out what you want to say. Do not expect to be able to submit your first draft. You will usually need to draft material more than once before it is ready. SWOT analysis can be used to identify and overcome problems, will give you confidence in areas that you are good at, and may be useful in setting personal milestones.

Adopt the structure given by your university and explain it in your introduction. Check with your supervisor and university in the early stages whether your interpretation of the structure is acceptable. In addition to your headings, you should guide the reader through it with clear 'signposting' (i.e. explaining at each stage the stage that has been reached and what you are going to discuss next). Finally, try to get your dissertation ready before the deadline to allow time for a final proofread as this will pay dividends.

Remember that a good research proposal shows examiners that you are competent to carry out the research effectively and ethically. Use your overall question to signpost examiners about your methodological stance, and use your literature to argue and justify your study and your methods.

Further reading

Becker, H (2007) *Writing for Social Scientists: How to Start and Finish your Thesis, Book or Article,* 2nd edition. Chicago, IL: The University of Chicago Press.
A classic text that provides a very readable and entertaining account of the writing process.

Locke, LF, Spirduso, WW and Silverman, SJ (2014) *Proposals That Work: A Guide for Planning Dissertations and Grant Proposals,* 6th edition. California: Sage.
Gives information on funding grant applications.

Offredy, M and Vickers, P (2010) *Developing a Healthcare Research Proposal: An Interactive Student Guide.* Oxford: WileyBlackwell.
Student-focused text.

Punch, K (2006) *Developing Effective Research Proposals,* 2nd edition. London: Sage.
Good book with more detail on writing proposals.

Thomas, D and Hodges, ID (2010) *Designing and Planning Your Research Project.* London: Sage.
More detail on writing proposals.

Walliman, NSR (2014) *Your Undergraduate Dissertation: The Essential Guide for Success.* London: Sage.
More tips on effective writing.

Useful websites

http://library.bcu.ac.uk/learner/writingguides/1.07.htm
Birmingham University Study Guide on how to write a research proposal.

http://www2.hawaii.edu/~gangnes/730ResearchProposalHowTo.htm
Hawaii University module (Econ 730) site: useful, with lots of links on proposal writing.

Conclusion

In this book we have presented a wide variety of material that will help you to undertake research literature searching and reviewing, research proposal writing and planning systematic reviews. The emphasis has been on helping you to gain underpinning knowledge, which you can then use for your final-year assignments or dissertations concerning project planning and literature reviewing. Planning research may seem an unlikely task for a student nurse, hoping soon to be a newly qualified staff nurse, but it should be remembered that the 'point' of these assignments is as much about developing transferable skills as it is about formulating research proposals.

In your new role, you will quickly be expected to take on clinical leadership roles, particularly if, as seems likely, you will quickly be expected to supervise Band 4 and other unregistered staff as one of only a few Band 5 nurses and above in a shift. Clinical leadership is about skills, attributes and personality, but it is first and foremost about excellent clinical practice, and in order to be able to identify excellent clinical practice, rather than simply operating on 'custom and practice', or 'we always do it like that', you need to have the knowledge to find and appraise evidence, including primary research reports and systematic reviews. These are skills that have been outlined in this book. They are important generic skills that you can apply to any aspect of clinical practice of your interest. As you become more senior it is likely that you will take on greater responsibilities than nurses have previously had, with greater autonomy, and even possibly independent prescribing rights: treatment decisions will be yours alone, and in order to make the correct choices for your patients you will need to be able to understand the studies that indicate different options. Also, patients are very well informed these days via the internet, and you will need to be able to evaluate the quality of information they present to you about their illnesses and treatments in order to be clinically credible to them. Will you be able to tell them why an article in a popular women's magazine, or an internet advert, is of less value in making treatment decisions than a Cochrane systematic review or National Institute for Health and Care Excellence (NICE) guidelines? After reading this book you should be able to.

The second element of this book is about planning research projects. Again, you may argue that you'll never be doing research yourself, but you will find as your career progresses that you are expected to undertake further qualifications as part of your work role, or in order to gain promotion. It is apparent from our experience in education that many candidates for Master's degrees have very little background in understanding and applying research methods effectively, and this puts them at a disadvantage compared to other professions that do have that background. We emphasise that it is not learning about research methods that is in itself important, but it is their application in the clinical setting, and this is why you are being asked to plan a project: to show that you understand the existing literature, potential study designs, methods of inquiry and ethical issues sufficiently well. It is also not beyond the realms of possibility that you might be involved with research studies taking place in your workplace, or want to investigate some aspect of clinical care and how to improve it in the future. Nursing will not build a research culture unless clinical nurses identify and investigate clinical questions, and you could be part of that future.

In the introduction we outlined how this book meets the Nursing and Midwifery Council (NMC) Standards for Pre-registration Nursing Education (NMC, 2010a) as well as its Essential Skills Clusters (NMC, 2010b) and the Quality Assurance Agency (QAA, 2001) subject benchmarks for nursing. We have reproduced these, to show how the knowledge and skills you have acquired in this book meet outcomes specifically related to the newly qualified nurse; the *italic* text indicates how they have been addressed.

NMC Standards for Pre-registration Nursing Education (NMC, 2010a)

Domain: Professional values

9. All nurses must appreciate the value of evidence in practice, be able to understand and appraise research, apply relevant theory and research findings to their work, and identify areas for further investigation.

We have discussed a range of research methodologies. Literature searching and project planning can help you to further your knowledge about nursing practice in your area.

Domain: Nursing practice and decision making

1. All nurses must use up-to-date knowledge and evidence to assess, plan, deliver and evaluate care, communicate findings, influence change and promote health and best practice. They must make person-centred, evidence-based judgments and decisions, in partnership with others involved in the care process, to ensure high quality care. They must be able to recognise when the complexity of clinical decisions requires specialist knowledge and expertise, and consult or refer accordingly.

Finding and reviewing literature will help you to make evidence-based judgements on best available care for your patients. Being able to identify best practice will allow you to recommend changes to what goes on in your area.

Essential Skills Clusters

The NMC Essential Skills Clusters (2010b) require a level of research literacy and skills with evidence.

Cluster: Organisational aspects of care

9. People can trust the newly registered graduate nurse to treat them as partners and work with them to make a holistic and systematic assessment of their needs; to develop a personalised plan that is based on mutual understanding and respect for their individual situation promoting health and well-being, minimising risk of harm and promoting their safety at all times.

(continued)

continued ... •

By entry to the register.
- Applies research-based evidence to practice.

Finding and reviewing literature will help you to make evidence-based judgements on best available care for your patients; being able to identify best practice will allow you to recommend changes to what goes on in your area.

16. People can trust the newly registered graduate nurse to safely lead, co-ordinate and manage care.

By entry to the register
- Bases decisions on evidence and uses experience to guide decision making.

Finding and reviewing literature will help you to make evidence-based judgements on best available care for your patients.

20. People can trust the newly registered graduate nurse to select and manage medical devices safely.

By entry to the register
- Works within legal frameworks and applies evidence-based practice in the safe selection and use of medical devices.

Finding and reviewing literature will help you to make evidence-based judgements on best available care for your patients.

Cluster: Medicines management

41. People can trust the newly registered graduate nurse to use and evaluate up-to-date information on medicines management and work within national and local policy guidelines.

You now know about NICE and Scottish Intercollegiate Guidelines Network (SIGN), as well as Cochrane and Joanna Briggs, and these are the bodies from which policy guidelines can be obtained. This indicates your clinical leadership responsibilities in this area.

By the second progression point
- Accesses commonly used evidence-based sources relating to the safe and effective management of medicine.

By entry to the register
- Works within national and local policies and ensures others do the same.

Benchmark Statement for Health Care Programmes

The QAA (2001) Benchmark Statement for Health Care Programmes indicates that in nursing the following are important in relation to research and evidence.

A1 Professional autonomy and accountability

The award holder should be able to:

- contribute to the development and dissemination of evidence-based practice within professional contexts.

Met by accessing and critiquing research evidence as well as developing proposals.

A4 Profession and employer context

The award holder should be able to:

- recognise the value of research and other scholarly activity in relation to the development of the profession and of patient/client care.

Met in this book by a greater understanding of research methods.

- recognise the need for changes in practice from best available evidence.

Met by accessing and critiquing research evidence.

The study of nursing encompasses the following principle:

- the application of current knowledge and research to nursing practice across the health and illness continuum.

Met by accessing and critiquing research evidence.

B2 Formulation of plans and strategies for meeting healthcare needs

The award holder should be able to:

- use evidence-based options to facilitate patient choice and inform nursing interventions.

Met by accessing and critiquing research evidence.

B3 Practice

The award holder should be able to:

- conduct appropriate activities skilfully and in accordance with best/evidence-based practice;
- apply evidence-based knowledge to inform nursing care decisions.

Both met by accessing and critiquing research evidence.

C1 Knowledge and understanding

The award holder should be able to demonstrate:

- understanding of the key concepts of the disciplines that underpin the education and training of all healthcare professionals, and detailed knowledge of some of these. The latter would include a broad understanding of:
  - health and social care philosophy and policy, and its translation into ethical and evidence-based practice.

Met by accessing and critiquing research evidence.

(Continued)

(Continued)

C2 Associated skills

The award holder should be able to:

Information gathering
- seek out research-based evidence related to specific client groups;
- show an ability to gather and evaluate evidence and information from a wide range of sources;
- show an ability to use methods of enquiry to collect and interpret data in order to provide information that would inform or benefit practice.

Problem solving and data collection and interpretation
- analyse, interpret and assess the value of evidence to inform problem solving.

Met by accessing and critiquing research evidence.

Information technology
- access healthcare research and literature databases.

Met by literature searching

Teaching, learning and assessment

Generic and enabling skills

Programmes should be designed to facilitate students' acquisition of effective communication skills, team working, problem solving, the use of IT, research methodology and critical reasoning.

B Principles and concepts: application

The award holder should be able to:

- demonstrate critical understanding of research-based knowledge and the application to practice;
- use relevant theoretical and research evidence to inform a comprehensive, systematic assessment of the physical, psychological, social and spiritual needs of patients, clients and communities;
- critically evaluate research findings and suggest changes to planned care;
- use appropriate research and other evidence to underpin nursing decisions that can be justified, even when made on the basis of limited information.

Met by accessing and critiquing research evidence.

C Subject knowledge, understanding and associated skills

The award holder should be able to:

- demonstrate an understanding of research and other evidence and, where appropriate, apply findings to practice;
- critically evaluate research findings, suggest changes to practice and contribute to healthcare research to inform practice development.

Met by accessing and critiquing research evidence. Understanding demonstrated in literature review and proposal writing.

One key aspect that all student nurses are interested in is their employability. To that end we have mapped in Table 11.1 the key outcomes from the NHS Knowledge and Skills Framework (Department of Health, 2004) with suggested learning outcomes for undertaking a literature review and proposal module for nurses run by one of us (GW). This indicates that the skills you have learned by reading this book and undertaking your own modules are rated highly by the NHS for your work role as a newly qualified nurse and are transferable from higher education into the NHS.

Module learning outcomes	NHS Knowledge and Skills Framework dimension and level
Undertake a structured, systematic literature search relevant to the chosen topic using electronic databases	Communication 4c and e Service development 4b Quality 3c Production and communication of information and knowledge 4c, e, f, g, h, i, j Leadership 3a
Write a coherent research proposal, exploring methodological issues in study design	Service development 4b and c Leadership 3a Research and development 3a, b, c, d, e, f, g, h, i, j
Write a critical, integrated literature review on the chosen topic	Communication 3b, c, d Personal and people development 3a, b, c, d, e Quality 4b Data processing and management 2e Production and communication of information and knowledge 3a, c, d, g, i, j; 4e, f, h Leadership 2a Research and development 3a, b, c, e, f, g, h, i, j

Table 11.1: Literature searching and project planning outcomes mapped to the NHS Knowledge and Skills Framework

Above all, we hope you have enjoyed the book, passed your assignments, projects or dissertations, and are about to qualify for a demanding yet rewarding career as a nurse in your chosen field.

References

Alston, M and Bowles, W (1998) *Research for Social Workers.* St Leonard, NSW: Allen & Unwin.

Andersen, ML and Taylor, HF (2005) *Sociology: Understanding a Diverse Society.* Belmont, CA: Thomson Wadsworth.

Andrews, M, Day Sclater, S, Rustin, M, Squire, C and Treacher, A (eds) (2004) *Uses of Narrative.* New Brunswick, NJ: Transition.

Andrews, M, Squire, C and Tamboukou, M (eds) (2008) *Doing Narrative Research.* London: Sage.

Arksey, H and Knight, P (1999) *Interviewing for Social Scientists: An Introductory Resource with Examples.* London: Sage.

Aveyard, H (2010) *Doing a Literature Review in Health and Social Care,* 2nd edition. Berkshire: Open University Press.

Barbour, RS and Kitzinger, J (1999) *Developing Focus Group Research: Politics, Theory and Practice.* London: Sage.

Barthes, R (1972) *Mythologies.* New York: Hill & Wang.

Becker, H (1986) *Writing for Social Scientists: How to Start and Finish Your Thesis, Book or Article.* Chicago, IL: University of Chicago Press.

Becker, H (2007) *Writing for Social Scientists: How to Start and Finish Your Thesis, Book or Article,* 2nd edition. Chicago, IL: University of Chicago Press.

Berelson, B (1952) *Content Analysis in Communication Research.* New York: Free Press.

Bhaskar, R (1978) *A Realist Theory of Science,* 2nd edition. Atlantic Highlands, NJ: Humanities Press.

Bhaskar, R (1979) *The Possibility of Naturalism: A Philosophical Critique of the Contemporary Human Sciences.* Brighton: Harvester.

Bhaskar, R (1990) *Harré and His Critics.* Oxford: Blackwell.

Bloor, M, Frankland, J and Robson, K (2001) *Focus Groups in Social Research.* London: Sage.

Bottomore, TB and Rubel, M (1963) *Karl Marx: Selected Writings in Sociology and Social Philosophy.* Harmondsworth: Penguin.

Boyatzis, RE (1998) *Transforming Qualitative Information: Thematic Analysis and Code Development.* Thousand Oaks, CA: Sage.

Braun, V and Clarke, V (2006) Using thematic analysis in psychology. *Qualitative Research in Psychology,* 3: 77–101.

Braun, V and Clarke, V (2013) *Successful Qualitative Research: A Practical Guide for Beginners.* London: Sage.

Brink, P (1991) Issues of reliability and validity, in J Morse (ed.) *Qualitative Nursing Research: A Contemporary Dialogue.* London: Sage.

Bryman, A (2012) *Social Research Methods,* 4th edition. Oxford: Oxford University Press.

Caelli, K, Ray, L and Mill, J (2003) 'Clear as mud': toward greater clarity in generic qualitative research. *International Journal of Qualitative Methods,* 2 (2). Article 1. Available online at http://www.ualberta.ca/~iiqm/backissues/2_2/pdf/caellietal.pdf (accessed 4 July 2007).

Cartwright, N (2007) Are RTCs the gold standard? *Biosocieties,* 2: 11–20.

Chiang, C-Y and Sun, F-K (2009) The effects of a walking program on older Chinese American immigrants with hypertension: a pretest and posttest quasi-experimental design. *Public Health Nursing,* 26 (3): 40–248.

Clarke, M (2006) Part 1: Systematic review and meta analysis of quantitative research, overview of methods. Chapter 1, in C Webb and B Roe (eds) *Reviewing Research Evidence for Nursing Practice: Systematic Reviews*. Oxford: Blackwell Publishing, pages 1–8.

Clements, S and Foster, N (2008) Newspaper reporting on schizophrenia: a content analysis of five national newspapers at two time points. *Schizophrenia Research*, 98: 178–183.

Cooke, A, Smith, D and Booth, A (2012) Beyond PICO: the SPIDER tool for qualitative evidence synthesis. *Qualitative Health Research*, 22: 1435–1443.

Courtenay, M, Carey, N and Stenner, K (2009) Nurse prescriber–patient consultations: a case study in dermatology. *Journal of Advanced Nursing*, 65 (6): 1207–1217.

Crossley, M (2000) *Introducing Narrative Psychology: Self, Trauma and Construction of Meaning*. Buckingham: Open University Press.

Crossley, M (2007) Narrative analysis, in E Lyons and A Coyle (eds) *Qualitative Data Analysis in Psychology*. London: Sage.

Crossley, M and Crossley, N (2001) Patient voices, social movements and the habitus: how psychiatric survivors 'speak out'. *Social Science and Medicine*, 52: 1477–1489.

Crotty, M (1998) *The Foundations of Social Research: Meaning and Perspectives in the Research Process*. London: Sage.

Culley, L, Hudson, N and Rapport, F (2007) Using focus groups with minority ethnic communities researching infertility in British South Asian communities. *Qualitative Health Research*, 17: 102–112.

Curtis, EA and Redmond, R (2007) Focus groups in nursing research. *Nurse Researcher*, 14 (2): 25–37.

Daly, J, Willis, K, Small, R, Green, J, Welch, N, Kealy, M and Hughes, E (2007) A hierarchy of evidence for assessing qualitative health research. *Journal of Clinical Epidemiology*, 60 (1): 43–49.

Data Protection Act (1998) Available online at www.opsi.gov.uk/Acts/Acts1998/ukpga_19980029_en_1 (accessed 20 April 2010).

David, M (2006) Editor's introduction, in *Case Study Research: Sage Benchmarks in Social Research Methods*, vol. 1. London: Sage.

Davies, M (1997) Shattered assumptions: time and the experience of long-term HIV positivity. *Social Science and Medicine*, 44: 561–571.

Davies, MB (2007) *Doing a Successful Research Project: Using Qualitative or Quantitative Methods*. Basingstoke: Palgrave Macmillan.

Day, C, Carey, M and Surgenor, T (2006) Children's key concerns: piloting a qualitative approach to understanding their experience of mental health care. *Clinical Child Psychology and Psychiatry*, 11: 139.

Delamont, S, Atkinson, P and Parry, O (2004) *Supervising the PhD: A Guide to Success*, 2nd edition. Buckingham: Open University Press.

Denscombe, M (2007) *The Good Research Guide for Small-Scale Social Research Projects*, 3rd edition. Buckingham: Open University Press.

Department of Health (2001) *National Service Framework for Older People*. London: HMSO.

Department of Health (2004) *NHS Knowledge and Skills Framework*. Available online at www.dh.gov.uk/en/Publicationsandstatistics/Publications/PublicationsPolicyAndGuidance/DH_4090843 (accessed 21 July 2010).

Department of Health (2005) *Research Governance Framework for Health and Social Care*, 2nd edition. Available online at https://www.gov.uk/government/publications/research-governance-framework-for-health-and-social-care-second-edition (accessed 20 March 2014).

Diamond, I and Jeffries, J (2001) *Beginning Statistics: An Introduction for Social Scientists*. London: Sage.

Donnan, PT (2000) Experimental research, in D Cormack (ed.) *The Research Process in Nursing*. Oxford: Blackwell Science.

Dunleavy, P (2003) *Authoring a PhD: How to Plan, Draft, Write and Finish a Doctoral Thesis or Dissertation*. Basingstoke: Palgrave Macmillan.

Elliott, J (2005) *Using Narrative in Social Research: Qualitative and Quantitative Approaches.* London: Sage.

Ellis, P (2013) *Evidence-Based Practice in Nursing*, 2nd edition. London: Sage/Learning Matters.

Epstein, I (2009) *Clinical Data-Mining: Integrating Practice and Research.* New York: Oxford University Press.

Epstein, I, Zilberfein, F and Synder, S (1997) Using available information in practice-based outcomes research: a case study of psycho-social risk factors and liver transplant outcomes, in EJ Mullen and JL Magnabosco (eds) *Outcome Measurement in the Human Services: Cross-Cutting Issues and Methods.* Washington, DC: NASW Press, pages 224–233.

Eysenck, HJ (1995) Problems with meta analysis. Chapter 6, in I Chalmers and DG Altman (eds) *Systematic Reviews.* London: BMJ Publishing Group.

Farquhar, C (with Das, R) (1999) Are focus groups suitable for sensitive topics? in RS Barbour and J Kitzinger (eds) *Developing Focus Group Research: Politics, Theory and Practice.* London: Sage.

Finch, J (1987) The vignette technique in survey research. *Sociology*, 21: 105–114.

Frank, A (1995) *The Wounded Storyteller: Body, Illness and Ethics.* Chicago, IL: University of Chicago Press.

Free, C, White, P, Shipman, C and Dale, J (1999) Access to and use of out-of-hours services by members of Vietnamese community groups in South London: a focus group study. *Family Practice*, 16 (4): 369–374.

Gibbs, GR (2007) *Analysing Qualitative Data.* London: Sage.

Giddens, A (1993) *New Rules of Sociological Method: A Positive Critique of Interpretative Sociologies*, 2nd edition. Cambridge: Polity Press.

Giddens, A (2006) *Sociology*, 5th edition. Cambridge: Polity Press.

Glaser, B and Strauss, A (1967) *The Discovery of Grounded Theory.* Chicago, IL: Aldine.

Gough, D, Oliver, S and Thomas, J (2012) *An Introduction to Systematic Reviews.* London: Sage.

Gray, DE (2004) *Doing Research in the Real World.* London: Sage.

Green, J and Hart, L (1999) The impact of context on data, in RS Barbour and J Kitzinger (eds) *Developing Focus Group Research: Politics, Theory and Practice.* London: Sage.

Green, G, Hayes, C, Dickinson, D, Whittaker, A and Gilheany, B (2002) The role and impact of social relationships upon well-being reported by mental health service users: a qualitative study. *Journal of Mental Health*, 11 (5): 565–579.

Green, G, Hayes, C, Dickinson, D, Whittaker, A and Gilheany, B (2003) A mental health service users perspective to stigmatisation. *Journal of Mental Health*, 12 (3): 223–234.

Gubrium, JF and Holstein, JA (2009) *Analysing Narrative Reality.* Thousand Oaks, CA: Sage.

Happel, B (2007) Focus groups in nursing research: an appropriate method or the latest fad? *Nurse Researcher*, 14 (2): 18–24.

Hart, C (2001) *Doing a Literature Search: A Comprehensive Guide for the Social Sciences.* London: Sage.

Hek, G and Moule, P (2006) *Making Sense of Research: An Introduction for Health and Social Care Practitioners*, 3rd edition. London: Sage.

Hemingway, P and Brereton, N (2009) What is a systematic review? Bandolier evidence based medicine series. Available online at www.medicine.ox.ac.uk/bandolier/painres/download/whatis/Syst-review. pdf (accessed 12 July 2010).

Heron, J and Reason, P (2006) The practice of co-operative inquiry: research 'with' rather than 'on' people, in P Reason and H Bradbury (eds) *Handbook of Action Research.* London: Sage.

Hinchman, LP and Hinchman, SK (1997) Introduction, in LP Hinchman and SK Hinchman (eds) *Memory, Identity, Community: The Idea of Narrative in the Human Sciences.* New York: State University of New York.

Hollis, S and Campbell, F (1999) What is meant by intention to treat analysis? Survey of published randomised controlled trials. *British Medical Journal*, 319 (7211): 670–674.

Howick, J (2009) Oxford Centre for Evidence-Based Medicine Levels of Evidence. Produced by Phillips, B, Ball, C, Sackett, D, Badenoch, D, Straus, S, Haynes, B, Dawes, M since November 1998. Updated by Howick, J, March 2009. Available online at www.cebm.net/index.aspx?o=1025 (accessed 13 July 2010).

Huberman, M and Miles, M (1998) Data management and analysis methods, in N Denzin and Y Lincoln (eds) *Collecting and Interpreting Qualitative Materials*. London: Sage.

Humphries, B (2008) *Social Work Research for Social Justice*. Basingstoke: Palgrave Macmillan.

Janis, IL (1982) *Groupthink*, 2nd edition. Boston, MA: Houghton Mifflin.

Khan, SK, Kunz, R, Kleijnan, J and Antes, G (2003) *Systematic Reviews to Support Evidence Based Medicine*. London: Royal Society of Medicine.

Kirby, S and McKenna, K (1989) *Experience, Research, Social Change: Methods from the Margins*. Toronto: Garamond.

Kitzinger, J (1994) The methodology of focus groups: the importance of interaction between research participants. *Sociology of Health and Illness*, 16 (1): 103–121.

Koch, T, Kralik, D, Eastwood, S and Schofield, A (2008) Breaking the silence: women living with multiple sclerosis and urinary incontinence. *International Journal of Nursing Practice*, 7 (1): 16–23.

Kralik, D, Price, K, Warren, J and Koch, T (2006) Issues in data generation using email group conversations for nursing research. *Journal of Advanced Nursing*, 53 (2): 213–220.

Krueger, RA (1994). *Focus Groups: A Practical Guide for Applied Research*. Thousand Oaks, CA: Sage.

Krueger, RA and Casey, MA (2000) *Focus Groups*, 3rd edition. Thousand Oaks, CA: Sage.

Kvale, S (1996) *Interviews: An Introduction to Qualitative Research Interviewing*. London: Sage.

Labov, W and Waletsky, J (1967) Narrative analysis: oral versions of personal experience, in J Helms (ed.) *Essays in the Verbal and Visual Arts*. Seattle, WA: University of Washington.

Layder, D (1993) *New Strategies in Social Research*. Cambridge: Polity Press.

Leki, I (1998) *Academic Writing: Exploring Processes and Strategies*. Cambridge: Cambridge University Press.

Lincoln, YS and Guba, EG (1985) *Naturalistic Inquiry*. London: Sage.

Lloyd Jones, M (2006) Part 2: Meta-synthesis and meta-study of qualitative research, overview of methods (Chapter 6), in C Webb and B Roe (2006) *Reviewing Research Evidence for Nursing Practice: Systematic Reviews*. Oxford: Blackwell Publishing, pages 63–72.

Ludema, JD, Cooperrider, DL and Barrett, FJ (2006) Appreciative inquiry: the power of the unconditional positive question, in P Reason and H Bradbury (eds) *Handbook of Action Research*. London: Sage.

Macdonald, J (2003) *Using Systematic Reviews to Improve Social Care*, SCIE Report No. 4. London: Social Care Institute for Excellence.

Mair, M (1989) *Between Psychology and Psychotherapy*. London: Routledge.

Maxwell, JA (1996) *Qualitative Research Design: An Interactive Approach*. Thousand Oaks, CA: Sage.

McCulloch, G (2004) *Documentary Research in Education, History and the Social Sciences*. London: Routledge Falmer.

Merton, RK, Fiske, M and Kendall, P (1990) *The Focused Interview*, 2nd edition. New York: Free Press.

Michell, L (1999) Combining focus groups and interviews: telling how it is, telling how it feels, in RS Barbour and J Kitzinger (eds) *Developing Focus Group Research*. London: Sage.

Miles, MB and Huberman, AM (1994) *Qualitative Data Analysis: An Expanded Sourcebook*, 2nd edition. London: Sage.

Moher, D, Hopewell, S, Schulz, KF, Montori, V, Gøtzsche, PC, Devereaux, PJ, Elbourne, D, Egger, M and Altman, DG, for the CONSORT Group (2010) CONSORT 2010. Explanation and elaboration: updated guidelines for reporting parallel group randomised trial. *BMJ*, 340: c869.

Morgan, DL (ed.) (1993) *Successful Focus Groups: Advancing the State of the Art*. London: Sage.

Morgan, DL (1997) *Focus Groups as Qualitative Research*, 2nd edition. London: Sage.

Morgan, DL (1998) *Planning Focus Groups*. Thousand Oaks, CA: Sage.

Moule, P and Goodman, M (2009) *Nursing Research: An Introduction*. London: Sage.

Mulrow, CD (1995) Rationale for systematic reviews (Chapter 1), in I Chalmers and DG Altman *Systematic Reviews*. London: BMJ Publishing Group.

Nardi, PM (2006) *Doing Survey Research: A Guide to Quantitative Methods*. Boston, MA: Allyn & Bacon.

National Institute for Health and Clinical Excellence (NICE) (2009) *The Guidelines Manual 2009*. Available online at www.nice.org.uk/aboutnice/howwework/developingniceclinicalguidelines/clinicalguidelinedevelopmentmethods/GuidelinesManual2009.jsp (accessed 12 July 2010).

National Patient Safety Agency (2009) *About Us. How We Work.* Available online at www.nres.npsa.nhs.uk (accessed 27 May 2010).

National Patient Safety Agency (2010) *Defining Research.* Available online at www.nra.nhs.uk (accessed 27 May 2010).

Neuman, WL (2006) *Basics of Social Research: Qualitative and Quantitative Approaches,* 2nd edition. Boston, MA: Allyn & Bacon.

NHS Centre for Reviews and Dissemination (2006) Undertaking systematic reviews of research on effectiveness, CRD Report 4. York: The University of York NHS Centre for Reviews and Dissemination.

NMC (2010a) *Standards for Pre-registration Nursing Education.* London: NMC.

NMC (2010b) *Essential Skills Clusters for Pre-registration Nursing Programmes.* London: NMC.

Nuremberg Code (1949) *Trials of War Criminals Before the Nuremberg Military Tribunals under Control Council Law No. 10, Vol. 2, pp. 181–182.* Washington, DC: US Government Printing Office. Available online at https://owlspace-ccm.rice.edu/access/content/user/ecy1/Nazi%20Human%20Experimentation/Pages/the%20code.html (accessed 27 May 2010).

O'Leary, Z (2004) *The Essential Guide to Doing Research.* London: Sage.

Owen, S (2001) The practical, methodological and ethical dilemmas of conducting focus groups with vulnerable clients. *Journal of Advanced Nursing,* 36 (5): 652–658.

Parahoo, K (2006) *Nursing Research: Principles, Process and Issues,* 2nd edition. Basingstoke: Palgrave Macmillan.

Parker, I (1992) *Discourse Dynamics: Critical Analysis for Social and Individual Psychology.* London: Routledge.

Parton, N (2004) From Maria Colwell to Victoria Climbié: reflections on public inquiries into child abuse a generation apart. *Child Abuse Review,* 13: 80–94.

Payne, G and Payne, J (2004) *Key Concepts in Social Research.* London: Sage.

Peat, J (2002) *Health Science Research: A Handbook of Quantitative Methods.* London: Sage.

Philo, G (ed.) (1996) *Media and Mental Distress.* Harlow: Longman.

Plano Clarke, VL and Cresswell, JW (2008) *The Mixed Methods Reader.* London: Sage.

Potter, J and Wetherell, M (1987) *Discourse and Social Psychology: Beyond Attitudes and Behaviour.* London: Sage.

Punch, K (2005) *Introduction to Social Research: Quantitative and Qualitative Approaches.* London: Sage.

Quality Assurance Agency (2001) *Code of Practice for the Assurance of Academic Quality and Standards in Higher Education: Placement Learning.* London: Quality Assurance Agency.

Riessman, C (1993) *Narrative Analysis.* London: Sage.

Riessman, C (2007) *Narrative Methods for the Human Sciences.* London: Sage.

Ring, N, Ritchie, K, Mandava, L and Jepson, R (2011) *A Guide to Synthesising Qualitative Research for Researchers Undertaking Health Technology Assessments and Systematic Reviews.* Glasgow: NHS Quality Improvement Scotland (NHS QIS).

Robinson, FP (1970) *Effective Study,* 4th edition. New York: Harper and Row.

Robson, C (2011) *Real World Research,* 3rd edition. Oxford: Blackwell.

Rustin, M (2000) Reflections on the biographical turn in the social sciences, in P Chamberlayne, J Bornat and T Wengraf (eds) *The Turn to Biographical Methods in Social Science.* London: Routledge.

Sackett, DL, Strauss, SE, Richardson, WS, Rosenberg, W and Haynes, RB (1997) *Evidence Based Medicine: How to Practise and Teach EBM.* Oxford: Churchill Livingstone.

Sarantakos, S (2005) *Social Research,* 3rd edition. Basingstoke: Palgrave Macmillan.

Sarbin, TR (1986) *Narrative Psychology: The Storied Nature of Human Conduct.* Westport, CT: Praeger.

Saussure, F de (1983) *Course in General Linguistics.* London: Duckworth.

Scott, J (1990) *A Matter of Record: Documentary Sources in Social Research.* Cambridge: Polity Press.

Scottish Executive (2003) *Focus Groups with Minority Ethnic Communities.* Edinburgh: The Stationery Office.

Scourfield, J (2001) Interviewing interviewers and knowing about knowledge, in I Shaw and N Gould (eds) *Qualitative Research in Social Work.* London: Sage.

Sharp, J (2009) *Success with Your Education Research Project.* Exeter: Learning Matters.

Silverman, D (2013) *Doing Qualitative Research,* 4th edition. London: Sage.

Sim, J (1998) Collecting and analysing qualitative data: issues raised by the focus group. *Journal of Advanced Nursing,* 28 (2): 345–352.

Squire, C, Andrews, M and Tamboukou, M (2008) What is narrative research? in M Andrews, C Squire and M Tamboukou (eds) *Doing Narrative Research.* London: Sage.

Strauss, A and Corbin, J (1998) *Basics of Qualitative Research: Techniques and Procedures for Developing Grounded Theory.* London: Sage.

Thierfelder, C, Tanner, M and Bodiang, C (2005) Female genital mutilation in the context of migration: experience of African women with the Swiss health care system. *European Journal of Public Health,* 15 (1): 86–90.

Thurlow-Brown, N (1988) The Curate's Egg. Unpublished conference paper, North East Essex Mental Health Trust.

Tilling, K, Sterne, J, Brookes, S and Peters, TN (2005) Features and designs of randomized controlled trials and non-randomized experimental designs (Chapter 5), in A Bowling and S Ebrahim (eds) *Handbook of Health Research Methods: Investigation, Measurement and Analysis.* Milton Keynes: Open University Press.

University of Plymouth, Faculty of Health (2009) *Student Ethics Committee Guidelines and Application Form.* Plymouth: University of Plymouth.

Vaughn, S, Schumm, JS and Sinagub, J (1996) *Focus Group Interviews in Education and Psychology.* Thousand Oaks, CA: Sage.

Vissandjeé, B, Abdool, S and Dupéré, S (2002) Focus groups in Rural Gujarat, India: a modified approach. *Qualitative Health Research,* 12 (6): 826–843.

Walliman, N (2006) *Social Research Methods.* London: Sage.

Weissberg, R and Buker, S (1990). *Writing Up Research.* Englewood Cliffs, NJ: Prentice Hall.

Wilks, T (2004) The use of vignettes in qualitative research into social work values. *Qualitative Social Work,* 3 (1): 78–87.

Williamson, GR (2001) Does nursing need an ethical code for research? *NT Research,* 6 (4): 785–789.

Williamson, GR (2003) Misrepresenting random sampling? A systematic review of research papers in the *Journal of Advanced Nursing. Journal of Advanced Nursing,* 44 (3): 278–288.

Williamson, GR and Prosser, S (2002) Action research: politics, ethics and participation. *Journal of Advanced Nursing,* 40 (5): 587–593.

Williamson, GR, Collinson, S and Withers, N (2007) Patient satisfaction audit of a nurse-led lung cancer follow-up clinic. *Cancer Nursing Practice,* 6 (8): 31–35.

Williamson, GR, Callaghan, L, Whittlesea, E and Heath, V (2010a) Improving student support using placement development teams: staff and student perceptions. *Journal of Clinical Nursing,* 20: 828–836.

Williamson, GR, Jenkinson, T and Proctor-Childs, T (2010b) *Contexts of Contemporary Nursing,* 2nd edition. Exeter: Learning Matters.

Wong, PTP (2005) *How to Write a Research Proposal.* Available online at www.meaning.ca/articles/print/writing_research_proposal_may02.htm (accessed 4 May 2005).

World Medical Association (2013) Declaration of Helsinki: ethical principles for medical research involving human subjects. *Journal of the American Medical Association,* 310 (20): 2191–2194.

Yin, R (2009) *Case Study Research: Design and Methods,* 4th edition. London: Sage.

Zeller, R (1993) Focus group research on sensitive topics: Setting the agenda without setting the agenda, in DL Morgan (ed.) *Successful Focus Groups: Advancing the State of the Art.* London: Sage.

Index